Dr Nick Fuller is an internationally recognised health expert who has worked in both corporate and academic settings. He is currently responsible for the clinical research program within the Boden Initiative, located within the Charles Perkins Centre at the University of Sydney. He is also the director of clinical trials within the Department of Endocrinology at Royal Prince Alfred Hospital. Dr Fuller is a leading obesity researcher in Australia and has university degrees in exercise physiology, nutrition and dietetics, and a doctorate in obesity and weight management. He is a father of two children. For more information visit feedingfussykids.com and intervalweightloss.com.

T0356473

Also by Dr Nick Fuller

Interval Weight Loss
Interval Weight Loss for Life
Interval Weight Loss for Women

HEALTHY PARENTS, HEALTHY KIDS

Dr Nick Fuller

PENGUIN LIFE

UK | USA | Canada | Ireland | Australia
India | New Zealand | South Africa | China

Penguin Life is part of the Penguin Random House group of companies
whose addresses can be found at global.penguinrandomhouse.com

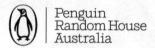

Penguin
Random House
Australia

First published by Penguin Life in 2024

Copyright © Nick Fuller 2024

The moral right of the author has been asserted.

All rights reserved. No part of this publication may be reproduced, published, performed in
public or communicated to the public in any form or by any means without prior written
permission from Penguin Random House Australia Pty Ltd or its authorised licensees.

The information contained in this book is provided for general purposes only. It is not
intended for and should not be relied upon as medical advice, nor is it intended to dictate
what constitutes reasonable, appropriate or best care for your child. The publisher and
author are not responsible for any specific health or allergy needs that may require medical
supervision. If you have underlying health problems, or have any queries about the
information in this book, you should contact a qualified medical, dietary or other
appropriate professional. Always discuss any concerns or questions about the health
and wellbeing of your child with a qualified healthcare professional.

Cover photography by OatmealStories / Getty Images
Cover design by Louisa Maggio © Penguin Random House Australia Pty Ltd
Typeset in 12.5/17 pt Adobe Garamond Pro by Midland Typesetters, Australia

Printed and bound in Australia by Griffin Press, an accredited
ISO AS/NZS 14001 Environmental Management Systems printer

A catalogue record for this
book is available from the
National Library of Australia

ISBN 978 0 14379 111 9

penguin.com.au

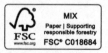

MIX
Paper | Supporting
responsible forestry
FSC® C018684

We at Penguin Random House Australia acknowledge that Aboriginal and Torres Strait
Islander peoples are the Traditional Custodians and the first storytellers of the lands on
which we live and work. We honour Aboriginal and Torres Strait Islander peoples'
continuous connection to Country, waters, skies and communities. We celebrate
Aboriginal and Torres Strait Islander stories, traditions and living cultures;
and we pay our respects to Elders past and present.

For my two beautiful boys, Jude and Jonas

CONTENTS

PROLOGUE

This book will change things for you. Maybe you've picked it up because you're worried about providing your child with a balanced diet, or maybe you're concerned about your own health. Many parents find that they put on a few kilos after their child is born – and this doesn't only apply to mums. Dads also struggle with their weight, despite their bodies not going through the same physical challenges of pregnancy and childbirth. Perhaps you've struggled with your health for your entire life, and you don't want your kids to experience the same challenges. Whatever your reason, this book can help, and by following the advice it contains, your whole family will benefit. It will provide you with the tools to set your child up for a healthy future, while also helping you as a parent get back on track to feeling healthier and full of energy. After all, healthy parents and healthy kids go hand in hand.

For parents, often the biggest challenge is knowing what foods you should provide your children, particularly if you have a picky eater. I am a father, so I know firsthand how fussy children can be, even more so at the end of the day when they are feeling shattered. We also live in a society where companies seek to profit from what we feed our kids, pushing incorrect and damaging advice on us and them. There is also an unending stream of advice, much of it outdated or plain old wrong.

Often the food habits of a parent are a blend of all the mixed food messages that they have received over the years, many of which were founded in misinformation. The science is clear and we have more access to information than ever before, but as a healthcare professional, I meet people every day who follow food concepts that are not based on science or that are many decades out of date. And these people, some of whom are now parents themselves, are passing on this misguided food advice to the next generation.

Your children will learn from what you do and eat; this goes for all facets of life, but none more so than what is placed in front of them at the dining table. You hold the keys to your child's food future.

Many parents see mealtimes as an opportunity to fill 'em up and get 'em out, which teaches your child that food is all about being 'fast' and unintentionally promotes a set of food-related behaviours that research tells us lead to negative health outcomes. I realise that with the endless demands of modern life, mealtimes can feel like yet another repetitive chore to get through, but I'm going to give it to you straight: you wouldn't light up a cigarette in your child's mouth, and you wouldn't let your child drink a can of beer, because you know the damage that this does to them. Over time, processed Western food can be just as detrimental to a person's health as a cigarette or beer. Saving time or placating children by giving them processed food will simply lead to a new generation that struggles with obesity, diabetes, heart disease and other underlying health concerns. Breaking out of these lifelong food habits and ways of thinking is hard to do, which is why so many people don't.

This book will guide you in establishing new, healthier habits and, in doing so, help you provide the best start in life for your children by futureproofing their diet and relationship with food.

It will do so in two ways: by introducing you to research-based and scientifically proven food facts; and by explaining how to apply these facts to achieve healthy outcomes for you and your family.

Some of you may be familiar with my work in the obesity and weight-loss field at the University of Sydney and Royal Prince Alfred Hospital. Rest assured that while this book will help *you* shift a few kilos, this is not a book about weight loss for children. It's the book that comes *before* that – the one that will help prevent the lifelong struggle with health and weight that many readers may have gone through as adults. It's a plan to help you form healthy habits that last a lifetime. It is never appropriate to fixate on a child's weight, and doing so will inevitably cause damage. Despite what you may have read online or been advised by others, body weight should never be the focus for children unless they are underweight and not getting enough nutrition. Instead, the focus should be on forming healthy habits which will then translate to an optimum body weight throughout their life.

As a leading scientist at the forefront of obesity research, I can tell you that obesity and weight gain are multifactorial, complex problems, and they are extremely challenging to address. Prevention is always easier than treatment, and as a parent you can shape your child's future and prevent a lifetime of pain and suffering, both physically and mentally.

This book is about freedom, not about feeling bad. I will not ask you to spend hours slaving over the stove making collagen gummies for babies or Instagram-worthy bento boxes for toddlers. It's a whole family approach, a practical guide to help you do your very best for your own health, and for the person you love most in the world: your child.

INTRODUCTION

The first 2000 days of a child's life – from conception to five years of age – offer a crucial window of opportunity for their health. These important days are a critical time of growth and development for your child's brain, body and immune system. It is when the foundations of your child's lifelong health are built.

Children absorb everything you expose them to and show signs of accelerated learning when they are under five years of age. During this crucial period, it is not only the neuronal connections in your child's brain that you're influencing with the experiences you provide for them, but also the entire body. The brain is intricately connected to our hormonal, metabolic, gastrointestinal, immune, cardiovascular, musculoskeletal and nervous systems. Think of the brain as a central computer that controls all the body's functions. What your child 'learns' during the first 2000 days of their life affects not only the brain but also the bodily systems to which the brain is connected.

Research clearly shows that a poor lifestyle during this critical stage may result in lifelong consequences for your child's health and wellbeing, including damage to their growing brain, an ongoing struggle with their weight, and major health concerns such as heart disease, type 2 diabetes and mental illness. While the first 2000 days are a golden opportunity for those with very small children, parents of older kids should take heart; science has repeatedly shown that many of the negative health impacts that your child might have been exposed to can absolutely be reversed by making the right dietary and lifestyle choices from here on out.

A healthy lifestyle is built on strong foundations of nutrition, physical activity and sleep. These factors play an essential role in your child's ability to grow, learn and thrive. Getting it right from the start will help ensure your child doesn't have an ongoing struggle with their health for years to come.

Our attitudes around nutrition and what we should consume are often influenced by what our parents taught us about food when we were children, which was based on the information available at the time. This means that a forty-year-old parent today may be passing on food habits rooted in 1980s research. That was when food fads made their dramatic entrance, including the likes of fat-free, low-carb and convenience packaged food. We now know that some of the information from that period is incorrect and many of these food fads do more harm than good when it comes to our health.

Let's take fat as an example. By the 1980s, several uncontrolled research studies emerged pointing to the dangers of high fat consumption leading to heart disease. Suddenly, a frenzied trend followed, with people actively reducing the amount of fat in their diet. This is certainly no bad thing in moderation, but it was a pendulum swing in the opposite direction. Food companies, capitalising on this new trend, started replacing fat additives with different types of sugar. The advertising that accompanied these products proudly declared that their product was 99 per cent fat free. They became 'diet' foods because they sounded like healthier options, but what the packaging failed to mention was the 90 per cent increase in added sugar.

Health-conscious consumers started buying 'reduced fat' biscuits, unaware that they contained the same number of calories as the regular variety because they were loaded with extra sugars instead. The reduced-fat option wasn't limited to unhealthy snack food; it was used in nutritious food too. Low-fat yoghurt, for example, saw a significant increase in its 'added sugar' content. And what happened because of the development of these seemingly healthy options? We began to get unhealthier.

In the intervening decades, many food fads have come and gone – keto, high protein, no sugar and, of course, no carbs. The fads might have changed, but the misinformation – and the damage it causes – remains.

We have far more information on the best food for health nowadays, but most of us still find it difficult to make the right choices. For parents, this might be because of overly busy lives, food confusion due to contradicting advice and influences, fussy kids, or a general lack of education. The ultimate result is a continuation of the food-fad era and the compromised wellbeing of ourselves and our children, leading to generations of unhealthiness.

As parents, we are being attacked by what we see on the shelves at supermarkets. We are being attacked by the opinions we absorb from those around us. We are being attacked by the information we see online and on social media. And the only way to defend your family is to become truly informed and knowledgeable, armed with research-led facts.

Moving forward

The good news is that this book can help you sort out food facts from fiction. As a qualified expert in my field, I'm here to give you advice that isn't linked to trends, marketing or product bias. All you will get from me is an explanation of clinically proven guidance about what you should be eating and what you should be feeding your children to give them the best possible chance in life. For many readers, this will require starting fresh and unlearning everything you've been told. That can certainly be a challenge! But remember, as a parent it's never too late to start again. And you've already taken the first step simply by picking up this book.

This whole family approach is based on six key principles. These principles reinforce and build upon the foundations of nutrition, physical activity and sleep: the essential ingredients for a healthy lifestyle. By applying them within your household, your family will learn new habits that stick. For parents, it will help you overcome the biological protections your body puts in place to hold on to excess weight and the evolutionary barriers that make it hard to manage your health and weight in our modern-day environment. For your children, it involves:

- Programming their body's set point – the weight their body is used to and most comfortable at – in a healthy range.
- Overcoming food fussiness.
- Eating wholesome, nutritious foods that are filling and tasty, allowing them to get the nutrition they need to grow and flourish.
- Giving them freedom to relax and enjoy the modern-day environment for what it is, so that they can enjoy the pleasures of readily available food.
- Being flexible and changing the plan to suit specific individual needs, such as coeliac disease, dairy intolerance and vegetarianism.
- Encouraging play that they enjoy and that becomes part of their daily life.
- Developing a healthy relationship with screens.

It does not involve:

- Depriving your child of food.
- Calorie counting, following set meal plans, or weighing out portions of foods for each meal.
- Setting a weight goal for your child.
- Complex cooking that requires you to track down an abundance of ingredients for each meal or locate obscure ingredients in supermarkets or health food stores.
- Cutting out any major food types.
- Creating food waste by using impractical ingredients.
- Cooking annoying or time-consuming recipes.
- Adopting a routine that is not sustainable or enjoyable.

Rest assured that by embracing the six principles of this program, you are choosing to follow a research-based lifestyle plan that will benefit the whole family. You'll improve your own health while helping your kids establish a positive relationship with food, exercise and sleep that will set them up for life.

The six steps to success

The first principle: *Health, not weight*

Weight loss will never be the focus when it comes to overall health. This can be hard for some people to action, and it might require you to shift your mindset, but it is imperative you do so for your child's sake. The healthy habits you develop and model for your family will ensure that your child has a naturally optimum body weight throughout their life.

The second principle: *Reach for nature first*

You will learn how to train your child's brain to appreciate 'nature's treats' and overcome the food fussiness that every parent knows so well. 'Nature's treats' are fresh foods consumed in their natural state, which are always a much better option than packaged, processed and fast food often containing a whole host of sugary and fatty additives. Some examples of nature's treats include raspberries, watermelon, honey and nuts.

The third principle: *The full rainbow*

You will focus on getting your child to eat more food, not less, with a focus on variety. Simple, whole foods are the most satisfying and nutritious of all foods, so it is important that your family's diet includes plenty of fruits, whole grains, nuts, dairy, fish, beans, and vegetables of all colours. No food types are eliminated.

The fourth principle: *Mealtime, feelin' fine*

You will start making a habit of sitting down at the dinner table and eating meals together as a family. Involving your child or children in meal preparation and serving is a great way to get them used to and invested in the routine. By doing so you will teach them the social benefits of eating together, as well as helping improve their innate appetite regulation by slowing down the family mealtime.

The fifth principle: *Play every day*

You will create opportunities for your child to play every day. By incorporating movement into your family's daily lifestyle, you will help your child learn that regular physical activity is an essential part of our health and wellbeing. You will also focus on offering a variety of activities to expose them to different environments.

The sixth principle: *Screen time showdown*

Overexposure to screens can cause a whole host of problems for your child's health and sleep. You will be required to model healthy tech habits, such as turning off all technology for two hours before bedtime and eliminating all forms of technology from the bedroom. For older children and teens, this will involve creating a plan together, so they feel in control of their choices. The evening time will instead be used to engage in activities such as reading, sport, going for family walks or other hobbies.

These principles might seem overwhelming at first; change is always difficult, particularly if you've been doing the same thing for years or even decades. But I assure you that by taking these principles to heart, one step at a time, you will improve the health of your whole family and set your kids up for life.

PART 1

PARTE

CHAPTER 1

HEALTH, NOT WEIGHT

As a parent, it's often hard to know whether you're doing the right thing, particularly when it comes to your child's growth and development during the first two years of their life. You take your child for their regular check-ups where the doctor or nurse jots down some measurements and then plots those weights, circumferences and lengths on various charts. For a few parents it might be stress free, especially if your child's line is plotting within the target range. But for many of you this process can be daunting, particularly if you're told that your child's measurements have fallen off the chart and that something needs to be done to correct it. This is particularly common when it comes to weight.

The key to understanding our weight is a concept known as our 'set point'. Everyone has a set point – the weight at which your body is most comfortable, and the weight that you are most likely at now. This set point is programmed in the early years of life, during the first 2000 days. It doesn't mean you can't change a person's lifelong weight trajectory. But the research shows that it's a lot easier if emphasis is placed on the first 2000 days. Your child's weight during their infant and toddler years can influence their weight trajectory later in life. Children who are overweight by the time they turn two are at greater risk of carrying that extra weight – and the potential health issues it might create – throughout adulthood. If the problem persists by the time they reach adolescence, the data shows that 80 per cent of children will struggle with their weight for the rest of their life.

But, as I emphasised earlier, this doesn't mean you should focus on your child's weight. Weight loss will never be the goal. Instead, you should embrace the six healthy habits in this book to ensure your child's set point is naturally programmed at the optimum point, to set them up for a lifelong healthy weight. By doing so, you'll also build the foundations for good health that will be retained over a lifetime.

Our genes

We all like to use our genes as a scapegoat when it comes to our struggle with weight. But the truth is, genetics are not to blame for the increasing rate of obesity we see today. Our genes haven't collectively changed over time. Our genetic material – better known as our DNA – contains tens of thousands of different genes. However, only 2 per cent of our total DNA contains genes that might mutate and result in obesity or other disease. Of the other 98 per cent, a small part controls how these genes are turned on or off, and the rest have no known function. For example, regular consumption of fast food can interact poorly with genes related to obesity, effectively turning these genes 'on'. For people with a genetic predisposition to obesity, eating a healthy diet can help avoid switching on these obesity genes.

Even if you or your child has a genetic predisposition to obesity, it is not an inevitable fate. Many people who carry 'obesity genes' do not become overweight, and healthy lifestyles can counteract these genetic effects.

How much weight gain is expected during pregnancy?

As this is a book about setting up the next generation for life, it is important that we start with pregnancy. Irrespective of your weight when you fall pregnant, it is healthy and normal to put on weight during pregnancy. So don't panic when you see the number on the scale start to change – you're growing a person!

If you were overweight at the time of conception (clinically diagnosed as BMI 25 kg/m^2 or above), then a weight gain of 9 kg over the nine-month period is healthy and expected. And of course, if you are pregnant with twins, this will be approximately double – a 20 kg weight gain over the nine-month period. If you fell pregnant when you were in what is considered a healthy weight range, then you can expect an even greater weight gain during pregnancy – approximately 12.5 kg, and you will gain most of this weight after 20 weeks from the date of conception. This is of course an average: gaining a few kilos more or less is nothing to panic about.

By the time you reach your due date, more than a third of the extra weight will come from your baby (approximately 3.3 kg), the placenta (0.7 kg) and amniotic fluid (0.8 kg). But your body will also have changed to help grow and nourish your baby, which accounts for the other two-thirds of your expected weight gain over the course of the pregnancy. There will be an increase in your breast size, uterus size, blood volume and body fluid, and you'll gain an extra 4 kg of fat to give you the energy you'll need for breastfeeding once your baby is born.

Most of the 9 to 12.5 kg weight increase that will occur during pregnancy will disappear in the first six months after the delivery of your child, without you actively trying to lose weight. Better yet, bin the scales for the nine months you are pregnant – they aren't helpful.

If you keep up your daily exercise and make healthy food and lifestyle choices (as outlined in this book), it doesn't matter how much weight you gain while you are pregnant. By making informed, sensible decisions about what you put in your body and how you treat it, then you can let your incredible body look after itself. This will ensure you deliver a healthy baby and that you maintain your own health during pregnancy and beyond.

Tracking your child's growth and development

Most of your child's brain development – 90 per cent of it – happens before they turn five. Therefore, it's important to monitor their growth and development regularly from the time they are born to the time they reach five years of age (when they typically start school). These regular checks ensure any potential issues are discovered early; it's much easier to fix them while your child is still growing and developing rather than later in life. Even if you think your child is tracking well, it gives you the opportunity to learn more about their growth and development and ensure nothing is missed. Scheduled health checks with your family doctor or your local Child and Family Health Centre should take place at key development stages in the first 2000 days of your child's life. As a general guide, this will happen at birth; a couple of weeks after birth; then at two, six, twelve and eighteen months; and then at two, three and four years of age.

Measuring your child's height, weight and head circumference can give a good indication of how your child is growing. Because children and adolescents are constantly growing, however, it's not always easy to know if your child is tracking appropriately for their age. It is never appropriate to apply the same measures for children as the ones we use for adults (such as BMI). Instead, your nurse or family doctor will use age-appropriate growth charts to track and interpret your child's growth and development. This is particularly relevant during the early stages of life, or when your child is less than two years of age.

Age-appropriate growth charts are typically split up into two categories: one for birth to two years of age, and another from two to eighteen years of age. Ideally, kids will stay within a certain range as they grow, meaning they have what is considered a healthy weight, height and head circumference for their age. However, these charts can cause a lot of anxiety and stress for parents, and they present their own challenges, particularly when it comes to tracking body weight during the early stages of life. A child less than two years of age is rapidly changing, and their growth is not always linear. Children learn to crawl and walk at different stages, and the rate at which their body weight increases will slow down when they begin to be more active, which can affect where they are tracking on a graph. Therefore, it is more important to assess the change in weight over time and to monitor trends in growth rather than panicking over a single measurement that might be an outlier. The same can be said for a child's height and head circumference. Don't get too hung up on one measurement, because it doesn't provide a meaningful assessment of your child's health.

It is quite common for a baby initially tracking between the 85th and 97th weight percentile to drop into a lower percentile once they start crawling and walking. So, despite what you might get told by a friend, colleague or family member, there is absolutely no need for concern if your child is tracking above the 85th percentile for weight – from birth to two years – providing you are following all the advice in this book to ensure you and your child have a healthy lifestyle. Your child's weight will correct itself as they start to crawl, walk and become more active. If you find yourself in a position where your child's weight is not below the

85th percentile after three months of walking alone, you should consider re-evaluating their current habits and your family habits, as outlined in later chapters. But whatever you do, don't start restricting the volume or type of food you are giving your child. Remember: the focus is health, not weight. Too often I hear of healthcare professionals, such as general practitioners and health-care nurses, who tell parents to start restricting their child's food intake; this is not correct advice. If it happens to you, I encourage you to seek a new doctor if possible.

Similarly, if your child is on the other side of the scale – if they're underweight, or below the 5th percentile – you might worry that your child's growth is stunted. Rather than jumping to any conclusions, it's important to talk to a paediatrician, who will advise if this is the case. If your child's growth is tracking in the right direction and they are growing over time, that's all that matters – even if they're not on the standardised chart. All children grow and develop at different rates.

A previous patient of mine, Jason, had recently become a father. He took his baby for his six-month milestone check-up. The maternal child health nurse advised Jason and his wife that their formula-fed son was visibly overweight and that overfeeding him had stretched his stomach, affecting his metabolism and leading to the baby demanding more food.

Shortly after this visit, Jason contacted me for advice as he was unsure that the nurse's advice to restrict his baby's meals was correct. Understandably, this conversation with the nurse had stirred up anxiety and shame for Jason and his wife.

The visit had also made them worried about solid food. As their son was now six months old, he was being fed purees in addition to formula. After taking their child's food history, the nurse told them that they shouldn't give him food pouches, because they contain fruit purée, which is high in sugar. Yet the pouches they were giving their boy were 100 per cent fruit and veg, with no added sugar.

Jason and his wife had not overfed their child; they'd simply been given incorrect information. I advised Jason that once his boy started moving – crawling and walking – his weight trajectory would correct itself and he'd likely return to the average percentile for his age.

As parents, their instincts about how much to feed their son were correct; he was regulating his calorie intake according to his needs. While not all food pouches are created equal and it's important to read the ingredients if you go down this route, the pouches Jason and his wife were providing were perfectly fine as they were 100 per cent fruit and veg, with no added ingredients. They were also giving their son a variety of solid foods and textures (different purée pouches, as well as finger foods such as pasta, avocado, chicken and berries), indicative of a well-balanced diet for his age.

Jason's son is now two years old and tracking in the 50th weight percentile for his age.

Body Mass Index (BMI)

We're a society fixated on numbers. So it's no surprise we use measurements and equations to track our weight. The most popular is BMI, a measure of our body weight-to-height ratio to ascertain whether someone is in a healthy body-weight range. However, this standard scale is intended for adults, and not for children and adolescents, whose bodies are still growing and changing.

Even for adults, BMI shouldn't be used as the single measure of what it means to be a healthy weight, because it fails to consider two critical factors related to body weight and health – body fat percentage and distribution – and it does not account for significant differences in body composition based on gender, ethnicity and age. Instead of relying on BMI alone, it's important to focus on measures that tell us where fat is distributed in the body, measuring weight circumference, waist-to-hip ratios and body fat to get a better understanding of health and risk. It's also important to consider other ways to measure your health and likelihood of disease, including levels of triglycerides (a type of fat found in your blood), blood cholesterol, blood glucose (sugar), blood pressure, heart rate and liver function.

Anna took her three-year-old daughter, Claudia, to their family GP because Claudia hadn't done a poo for five days.

Her regular doctor wasn't available, so Anna and Claudia saw another GP. But this GP didn't address Claudia's constipation; instead, they told Anna that Claudia was 'grossly overweight', it was all Anna's fault, and Claudia needed to go on a diet immediately. 'You're not going to like this,' the GP said to Anna, 'but you are hugely overweight too.'

Anna left the doctor's practice in tears (and with no solutions for her daughter's constipation). Having suffered body-image issues her whole life, Anna was savvy enough to know that a diet for a toddler was not the answer. Instead of following this bad advice, she contacted me, and I affirmed that she was doing the right things for Claudia: feeding her a wide variety of whole foods; not giving her the processed junk that toddlers *love* more than twice a week; and ignoring the scales.

Instead of focusing on Claudia's weight and food intake, we brainstormed how to include more playtime and reduce her screen time usage. I also assured Anna that toddlers can go several days without having a bowel movement, and that because Claudia had been unwell, her food intake had reduced significantly over the past week. As she started to feel better and resumed eating normally, her bowel movements became daily again.

Claudia's weight for her age has been changing significantly over the past two years, and at five years old she is now tracking midway between the 50th and 85th percentile.

Dieting

When parents believe their child's weight is tracking outside of the ideal healthy range, they sometimes go into 'dieting' mode because as adults this is how we've been taught to react. We are bombarded with mixed messaging and wrong information from the health and dieting industry, telling us that to achieve a healthy weight we must cut our food intake and omit certain foods or food groups from our diet. It seems like every day of the week a new food or food group is spotlighted as the cause of our weight problems. One minute it's fat, the next it's sugar, then it's carbs and now it's dairy. And if we're not careful, we're going to pass this misinformation and diet culture on to the next generation.

First, let's debunk a few food myths. Don't worry that certain fruits are 'fattening' because you've been told their sugar content is high. These are naturally occurring sugars, not the added kind you find in processed foods. Fruit is good for you and your child; it's packed with vitamins, minerals and fibre, which not only fills you up but is also good for your gut. Don't fear foods like bread, pasta and grains because you've been told that eating carbs leads to weight gain. Carbs have been a common scapegoat for weight problems for decades because when we eat them they store a lot of water in our body. Carbs are made up of many sugar units bundled together to form glycogen. And here's the interesting part: each gram of glycogen stored in your body is bound to 3 grams of water. So, as you can imagine, this can cause the number on the scale to jump up quite a bit. But it's no reason for concern, because this weight gain is simply an increase in your body's water content, not fat mass. In fact, carbs (the healthy type, not the sugar-coated processed stuff) are one of the key ingredients to good health.

Please, whatever you do, don't start restricting your child's food intake or put them on a diet. What might appear like a win at first can become detrimental later on. Research has shown that if you restrict the food intake of a young child, it might result in a lower weight at two years of age – but it leads to a higher weight by five years of age. What you're really doing is affecting your child's ability to metabolise food and their innate ability to regulate their food intake as they grow and develop, and guaranteeing a poor relationship with what they eat.

Sadly, diets aren't just an obsession for adults nowadays; they've become one for children and adolescents too. The multibillion-dollar dieting industry is doing its best to hook children into weight cycling – or 'yo-yo' dieting – early. Children and adolescents are exposed to social media, reality TV shows and magazines, just as we parents are, which can create a very un-realistic perception of what a healthy body weight looks like. This is particularly relevant for children who are old enough to be online – as a parent, you must make sure they understand that the images they see of people online are often snapped by a professional photographer or even edited by a smartphone app that pinches in their waist. Help your child understand that these images are fantasies, not real life. Everyone's body shape is different, and it is not healthy to try to look exactly like the people they follow on social media.

By role modelling healthy food consumption and educating your child on the dangers of dieting, you will ensure they don't have a lifelong struggle with their health and weight. Media literacy – knowing how to gauge the truthfulness of something you see in the press or online – is a crucial part of guiding your child's relationship with food and body image, especially as they grow older and might start wanting to replicate what they see on the screen.

Helping teens understand health versus weight

Many of you will have older children and teenagers who are in the midst of a different set of physical changes: puberty. This is a normal stage of development and it is entirely natural for their body to grow and look different as they undergo this major developmental process. But if you find yourself in a position where your adolescent is trying to change their weight, talk to them about it, honestly and openly. Identify the concerns they have about their weight and why these have come about. As a first step, you should help your child appreciate their body as it is – a piece of advice that applies to children of all ages. There is no one size fits all; people come in all different shapes and sizes, and overall health is more important than weight.

There are many reasons why your teenager may be feeling bad about their weight. Research shows that if you talk negatively about your own weight in front of your child, or worse still, you talk negatively about *their* weight in front of them, they're more likely to have body-image concerns and develop disordered eating behaviours themselves. Children learn fast, and they learn best by example. Be a positive role model and promote a healthy lifestyle for the whole family, rather than one that is tangled up in dieting and weight loss.

Social media may also be a contributing factor. Studies have shown that adolescents who spend more time on social media are less happy with their bodies and are at greater risk of developing disordered eating behaviours. Rather than trying to actively limit their online presence, start from a place of empathy and understanding; encourage them to unfollow accounts that leave them feeling bad or comparing their body to others and instead encourage them to seek out people who inspire them, make them laugh and help them feel empowered.

Your teen's concerns about their weight may also stem from issues they're having at school. Weight discrimination is a real phenomenon, and it is the number one reason why children and teenagers are teased at school. If you find out that your child is getting bullied or is receiving unkind comments from their peers, it's important to do something about it by discussing with relevant personnel at their school. Change starts from the top: there is demonstrably less weight discrimination and bullying in schools where teachers are proactive and willing to intervene, and at schools that address body weight in their anti-bullying policies.

Your teen's attitude towards weight won't change overnight. But if you keep up the message of health, not weight, and lead by example, you will be doing everything you can as a parent to set your child on the right path. Focus on establishing a healthy lifestyle for the whole family by changing those everyday behaviours that have a strong impact on health and wellbeing, which we'll get into throughout the rest of this book.

CHAPTER 2

REACH FOR NATURE FIRST

One of the biggest challenges kids throw at us is fussy eating. Fussy, picky, selective or choosy eating – however you name it – is very common in young children, and it usually peaks around three years of age. It refers to an unwillingness to eat familiar or new foods, and a lack of diet variety (typically less than 20 different foods in your child's diet). This can be a huge stress for parents, because if the fussiness persists, it can lead to poor growth and development, nutrient deficiencies and constipation. Plus, it's really annoying! But in fact, fussy eating is considered normal in young children, and as a parent you should expect it.

The literature shows that almost half of all children will go through a fussy eating period; it's a normal stage of development. Most kids are selective eaters, and it makes perfect sense, because it's this 'food fussiness' that ensured the survival of our ancestors, thousands of years ago. As humans, we rejected unfamiliar foods and bitter flavours – such as vegetables – to avoid ingesting potential toxins.

During our ancestors' time, food was hard to come by and calories were often scarce. To survive and procreate, humans learnt to seek out high-energy, palatable foods found in nature – foods that are packed with natural sugar, such as fruits and honey, and foods that are high in fat and protein, such as meat and nuts. Not only do they offer the best bang for buck from a calorie and nutrition point of view, but they also give us a natural rush, releasing all those feel-good chemicals in the brain every time we see and eat them.

Fast-forward a few hundred thousand years and it's a different story. Now we're spoilt for choice, but instead of taking advantage of nature's treats to fuel us, we rely on processed and 'fast' food that didn't previously exist. These fast foods also give us a high and release the same feel-good chemicals in the brain every time we see and eat them. Endorphins and dopamine are released in the brain's pleasure centre, the nucleus accumbens. The brain remembers this sense of satisfaction and triggers a positive response the next time we see the food. It's as if the brain has been hijacked.

But it's not only the high that makes it hard to stay away from these happiness-inducing foods; from an evolutionary point of view, we are wired to seek them out. Over time our genes haven't changed, but the food environment has. It has created an evolution-ary mismatch, where evolved traits that were once advantageous to ensure our survival have become harmful to us in modern-day life. In the case of food, our calorie-seeking brains were a useful trait when food was hard to come by, but not so much when we're submerged in a modern world saturated with food. We haven't evolved from these ancient survival circuits in the brain.

When it comes to your kids, it's easy to offer them food you know they will eat, but remember that what you feed them from a very early age will shape their lifelong food preferences. As parents, we need to be wary of wiring the next generation to get their food highs from fast and processed options loaded with added fats, sugars and salt. These foods are low in nutrition and very high in calories; they cause cravings and they can result in overconsumption due to a loss of portion control when eating them. It's worth pointing out, however, that not all processed foods are on an equal continuum. 'Processed' is a loose term, and it's important to read and understand ingredient labels to make healthier choices, which I'll get into later.

There is no doubt that this addiction to processed and fast food is vastly contributing to a generation of unhealthy children. Instead of letting your child become wired to rely on manufactured foods that are heavily processed, you'll need to teach them to rely on nutritious *everyday* foods in their natural state – fruits, vegetables, honey, nuts and seeds.

Setting the stage for healthy eating habits

While the genes that determine food fussiness have been passed on from our ancestors, it doesn't have to be our fate. I know it's hard – I have two very strong-willed sons, and getting them to eat different things is a struggle. But luckily there are five simple tips that make the process a whole lot easier to deal with your child's unwillingness to eat new foods:

Focus on a week's food intake, not a day's intake. It's hard to convince children or adolescents to try new things when they're tired from day care or stressed from the HSC. Give yourself – and them – a break and let them have an old favourite sometimes, even if it's not the healthiest option. Then focus on introducing different, nutritious foods on other occasions.

Avoid using food as a reward. Your child is not a dog!

Repeatedly provide nutritious foods in different ways. For instance, when introducing your child to avocado, try giving it to them on a cracker one day, or in a sandwich with Vegemite on another day, or even in a sushi roll.

Expose them to a wide variety of foods. Make sure you incorporate all the food categories in your family's meals throughout the week: grains, dairy, fruit, vegetables and lean protein.

Don't pressure them to eat. Instead, suggest they try something new and see if they like it. You might all be pleasantly surprised by the reaction!

The first step for you as a parent is becoming accustomed to exposing your child to lots of healthy food. Studies have shown that exposing children to a variety of foods before the age of two reduces fussy eating as they get older. One such study involved a large randomised controlled trial – the gold standard when it comes to research – that ran for five years. Mothers were randomly allocated to either an intervention group where they received support and education from healthcare professionals, or a control group, which included only self-directed access to the usual child health services. The researchers were interested in whether they could reduce food fussiness and promote healthy eating in children. The participating mothers were asked to report on the type and number of different foods their child had tried at 14 months of age. They were then asked to report on the type and number of different foods that their child liked at approximately four years of age. Children who were exposed to and tried a greater number of healthy foods – particularly fruit and vegetables – at 14 months of age were less likely to be fussy eaters at age four and their diets were much more varied. Children learn about food through exposure, specifically from seeing and tasting a variety of healthy foods. This increases their familiarity with a particular food, and, over time, they begin to accept and even like it.

So, as a parent, how do you do this? The best way to introduce your child to a wide variety of foods is by packing their lunchbox or plate with a bunch of different things, such as crackers with avocado, chopped fruit, pieces of cooked chicken or fish, cherry tomatoes, carrot or cucumber sticks, or a sandwich or wrap with avocado, cream cheese or similar. By including a bunch of options you're also less likely to tear your hair out because your child will eat at least some of what you have put on their plate.

Even though food refusal is extremely annoying, it's completely normal. You need to let your child decide how much they wish to eat. Learning how to deal with a child's food refusal early on is vital in reducing selective or picky eating later in life. As well as repeatedly offering your child nourishing, healthy food, it's important to not pressure them to eat it, to avoid using food as a reward (for example, promising them ice cream if they eat all their vegetables) and to avoid offering an alternative option if they don't eat what you first serve them. Research shows that if you do this when you first start introducing them to solids, it results in better dietary quality and healthier eating behaviours at five years of age. But it's not easy. As a parent myself, I can tell you that it requires a great deal of patience, and it's not a process you can speed up. Pressuring your kid into eating something is counterproductive and won't improve their fussiness. If they refuse a particular food, rather than pressuring them to eat it, try offering it again another time, perhaps in a different way. For instance, you could try minced meat in meatballs, spaghetti bolognaise, burgers or lasagne. And whenever possible, eat your meals with your child. You are the person they look up to. You are their role model and best pal. And, consequently, they'll copy everything you do. If you're eating the fruit and vegetables on your plate, they will eventually eat them too.

Every day will be different, so it's more important to focus on what your child is eating over the course of a week, rather than on any particular day. And remember, children are small human beings that require far smaller portions than adults. It's quite normal for them to be ravenous one day and then eat like a sparrow the next. Children are also very good at regulating their appetite, and this will be reflected by how much they eat on any given day. Millennial parents might recall being made to finish what was on their plate at dinner when they were children – don't do this! Research shows that parents who pressure their child to eat, who use food to calm or comfort their child, or who use food as a reward for their child will ultimately end up teaching them to eat for reasons unrelated to appetite. And this will have a long-term detrimental effect on their child's relationship with food and weight. So don't worry if your child rejects food or doesn't finish their meal – they are simply telling you that their energy stores are full and don't need to be replenished right now. Your task as a parent is to repeatedly provide a variety of nutritious and nourishing foods in a range of different ways to ensure your child has a healthy, varied diet. Children can decide for themselves when enough is enough.

It's also vital to remember that while a level of food fussiness or refusal is to be expected, you still need to keep an eye out for red flags when it comes to your child. Seek professional advice from a dietitian if their growth seems stunted, they're consistently refusing to eat certain textures, or if they avoid an entire food group (for example, dairy).

Rewiring your child's brain

The human brain reaches its full size in early adolescence, but it doesn't finish developing and maturing until your mid to late twenties. And it's the front of the brain, called the prefrontal cortex, that is one of the last parts of the brain to fully develop. The prefrontal cortex plays a key role in decision-making when it comes to food, which means there's plenty of time to rewire your child's brain and change their food choices.

The human brain contains neurons – approximately 100 billion of them. Each neuron has a long cable – several times thinner than a human hair – called an axon, and this is how signals travel from one neuron to another. These neurons form synaptic connections (up to 100,000) with each other, which allow them to communicate. This is the brain's 'wiring'. In your child's brain, this wiring is constantly changing and evolving. So, the good news is that you can effectively rewire your child's brain, even if right now they are a fussy eater and crying out for the fast and processed foods every day of the week. It isn't easy, and it does require some patience and perseverance – but it can be done.

As I mentioned at the start of this section, the part of your child's brain that we're particularly interested in is a specific area called the prefrontal cortex. Because the prefrontal cortex is responsible for decision-making, repeatedly providing your child with unhealthy food (for example, sugary, processed biscuits branded with your kid's favourite TV character) will only reinforce that decision-making process in their brain. In simplified terms, their neurons will communicate to each other that fast or processed food is 'good', and that is the food your child will gravitate towards. But the opposite also applies: regularly offering your child healthier food will train their brain to reach for those options instead. This means that as they grow up, your child will find it easier to make healthier decisions when it comes to food.

The best way to think of rewiring your child's brain is that it's like training a muscle. If you train it regularly, it will respond and strengthen over time. Repeatedly providing your child with healthy food will allow you to reshape their food choices over time so they start to enjoy nutritious food and ultimately become healthier and happier.

Forming new habits

You've done it – you've decided, 'No more. My whole family will be eating and living differently from now on.' Well done! But as you know, saying no and not giving in to your child's demands is challenging. However, making healthier choices doesn't mean saying 'no' all the time. Not allowing your child to eat what they love will only make them resentful and angry, and they might feel like they are missing out on what their friends are having. This sense of deprivation and resentment can then become engrained in their psychology, leading to an attitude as an adult of 'Stuff it, I'm going to do what I want,' which can result in a shift to the other end of the health pendulum and a return to poor food habits.

Let's consider a real-life example. Your child loves McDonald's, but you're trying to make sure the whole family is eating healthier. It doesn't mean they can *never* have food from there, but you will need to say no and be the unpopular parent most of the time. In the modern environment we are presented with these fast or processed food options all the time – rather than making the occasional appearance at a birthday or celebration, they have become part of our daily ritual. Try to break this habit; save Macca's for the occasional treat.

How long will it take to change my child's food choices?

Many parents have unrealistic expectations about the speed, ease and consequences of changing their child's behaviour. Irrespective of what you are trying to achieve, actual change takes time, effort and patience. This is particularly true when it comes to changing your child's food choices. Research has proven that it takes 66 days on average to create a new habit or to break an old one. Yes, that's right – it takes more than two months before a new behaviour becomes automatic, so it will be roughly eight weeks until your child starts to enjoy the berries and yoghurt instead of asking for a bakery or packaged treat.

After a couple of months of repeatedly offering your child nutritious and healthy food, you'll notice less resistance and more improvement in their behaviour as it relates to food. Keep a regular stock of nature's treats in your home, and offer them to your kid every time they're screaming out for the junk, and talk to them about the nutritional benefits and goodness found in such foods. Strawberries, berries, watermelon, mangoes, apples, nuts, tinned tuna and crackers, and honey (which you can give your child from 12 months of age), 100 per cent nut butter (from 4 to 6 months of age) or avocado on wholegrain toast all make great little snacks (more on that in the next chapter). The first 66 days are the hardest, but I am confident your child will be eating the bananas and fish soon!

Practising these behaviours regularly will make things easier for you too as your child will be more enjoyable to be around. Giving in to their food demands might seem like the quick fix to 'fill them up and get them out', but this short-term win will lead to long-term pain because they will always want the food you have allowed them on one occasion. Agitated children who do not get what they want are not easy to deal with or reason with. Research has also suggested that a poor diet can have a negative long-term impact on kids' behaviour.

Most importantly, remember that as their parent you need to model this eating behaviour for your child; don't let them see you snacking on a packet of chips when you offered them a handful of nuts instead. By embracing nature's treats yourself, your whole family will benefit.

CHAPTER 3

THE FULL RAINBOW

Food is the life force your child needs to grow and develop. During the first year of their life, their growth rate triples. In fact, it's the greatest period of growth for humans: length increases by approximately 17 centimetres at 6 months and by 25 centimetres at 12 months; and weight doubles in the first 5 months and triples by 12 months. But this is all dependent on good nutrition. Diet plays a major role in ensuring optimum growth; studies of 19-year-old adolescents in different countries have shown that those with poor nutrition ended up 20 centimetres shorter than their healthy-eating counterparts.

Your child's brain and head size also undergo huge changes during the first year of their life. Head circumference doubles in the first 12 months; it grows by 6 centimetres in the first 3 months, by 12 centimetres at 12 months, and by 16 centimetres at 3 years. And despite 70 per cent of one's brain size being reached by the age of three, it continues to grow well into adolescence. However, just like your child's height and weight, the growth and development of their brain is dependent on a steady supply of healthy and nutritious food. The brain is such a powerful organ that it consumes 50 per cent of the energy your child gets from the food they eat. If your child's brain doesn't get the energy it needs, it can negatively affect the growth of their brain, which can have a detrimental impact on your child's intelligence as they grow up. What you feed your child is a key pillar of their long-term success.

It's not just limited to physical development or growth; it applies to their mental development too. Research has consistently shown that a diet filled with 'junk' or processed food is associated with more mental illness and behavioural problems such as aggression, hyperactivity and mood swings. In fact, by repeatedly feeding your child a 'fast food' diet, you may be shrinking a part of their brain called the hippocampus, which plays a role in regulating their mood. There are many factors to consider when assessing a child's mood, but nutrition is one area where simple changes can have a big impact and we as parents can make the biggest difference.

To support the development of a healthy brain, body and immune system throughout childhood and adolescence, kids need to eat healthy, wholesome food – *the full rainbow*. Their diet should consist of dairy, meat, poultry, fish, cereals, whole grains, nuts, seeds, pulses, and fruits and vegetables of all colours. They don't need milk alternatives (except for the 5 per cent of children with an allergy to cow's milk), protein supplements, processed sugar or to avoid whole grains, nuts or dairy.

For parents

Your child's diet starts with you. Research has shown that we best use the energy from food in the morning – two and a half times more efficiently than in the evening. So don't be scared to load up your morning plate and let your food portions taper off throughout the day. It's better for long-term weight management, hence improving your overall health. Focusing on breakfast also kickstarts your metabolism and boosts your energy levels and alertness so you feel more energetic throughout the day. Quite simply, you can eat as much as you like at breakfast. If you are eating most of your food from breakfast through to lunch, and if dinner is your smallest meal, you are doing well. You should never deprive yourself of food, however, so if you're still hungry 10 minutes after eating, eat more, with a focus on extra salad and vegetables.

Hunger scale

The following scale is a very useful tool to help you become familiar with your appetite fluctuations, especially if you are only just now getting used to this way of eating. Start using a diary to record your hunger scale before and after meals. It is not the actual meal you need to record – there's no need for calorie counting or meal tracking – but rather what your appetite is doing and how it changes throughout the day.

-1	0	1	2	3	4
Full and uncomfortable	Not at all hungry	Satisfied	Slightly hungry	Somewhat hungry	Hungry

As I mentioned in chapter 2, forming a new habit takes time. It will take time to learn to gain an appreciation for how your appetite signals work in your body; this is not something that will happen overnight. If you notice that your hunger is high before meals at dinner ('3' or '4' on the hunger scale), you have a few tweaks to make when it comes to your diet and eating habits. This is particularly relevant if you have been in the same routine for years – perhaps skipping meals, eating little throughout the day, eating a lot of fast food, or having your biggest meal at dinner. The first step is simply to change your meal structure, to give yourself a chance of waking up hungrier in the morning. Over time, you should start to wake up in the '3' range of the hunger scale. If you wake up in the '4' range, you are doing very well.

The scale is also very useful for recording your hunger after eating a meal. Most of the time you should be at about '1' after eating, rather than '0' or '-1'. When you first make the switch to this way of eating, from big meals in the morning to smaller ones at the end of the day, you will find evenings the most challenging. Remember, this is not about depriving you (or your child) of food, so if you are still hungry after your first serve, go back for more! This is especially relevant for women during pregnancy and when breastfeeding. Your appetite will increase during these times, and this is normal and expected – after all, you're growing and feeding another person. But always stick to the 10-minute rule. That is, you should wait at least 10 minutes before you go back for more, as this is the amount of time needed for your 'appetite signalling' to work (that is, the time it takes for signals to be sent to your brain telling you whether you need more food). There is an exception: you can still eat as many salads and veggies as you like, and this applies to all meals. And even if you are pregnant or breastfeeding, you still need to follow the funnel plan of big to small meals throughout the day.

What foods should you avoid during pregnancy?

There is no need to become fixated on what you should and shouldn't eat during pregnancy, but there are a couple of high-risk foods that are better to avoid for the health of you and your baby. Some foods have a greater risk of containing harmful bacteria, such as listeria and salmonella, especially when they are raw. Foods to avoid include: raw eggs, meat and seafood; soft cheese; ready-to-eat luncheon meats (for example, deli meats); pâté; sushi; pre-prepared or packaged fruit, salads and sandwiches (including salad bars and smorgasbords); and raw beansprouts. It's best to avoid anything advertised as 'ready to eat'.

You can still enjoy a lot of foods, but you'll need to cook them first. Cooking food at risk of contamination kills off the harmful bacteria and makes it safe to eat (as is the case with eggs, soft cheese, seafood and meat). The other solution is to prepare food from scratch yourself, especially when it comes to things such as sushi, salads and sandwiches. And you can still have cheese! But it needs to be hard cheese – cheddar, for example – instead of soft cheeses such as brie, camembert, ricotta or feta. You can find a great infographic on foods to avoid at the Health Direct website: healthdirect.gov.au.

For kids

If you ensure your child eats nutritious meals regularly and you don't force them to eat all the food on their plate, they will be able to rely on their innate appetite signalling system for the rest of their life, without having to retrain it. Our appetite control gets disrupted if we are forced to eat when we aren't hungry, if we frequently skip meals, and if we often consume fast or processed food. A lack of appetite control can lead to overeating or making unhealthy food choices for instant gratification, ultimately leading to poorer overall health. If you find yourself in this position with your child, don't worry – it can be reversed. As your child grows and learns to understand their appetite, you can help them implement the hunger scale from as early as 10 years of age. But let's start by looking at your child's diet from the very beginning, when they're first born.

The first six months

Breastmilk or formula should be your child's only food source for the first six months of their life. A very small amount of mashed or pureed solids may be appropriate from the age of four months to help meet your child's additional nutritional needs. But it's best to avoid giving them regular cow's milk; a baby less than six months old cannot digest and absorb cow's milk as easily as breastmilk or formula due to its high protein content.

In the first few weeks of their life, your child will want to feed every 2 to 4 hours, so a total of 6 to 12 times over the course of 24 hours. This won't last forever! Overnight feeds aren't necessary after the age of 12 months. But the only way to know when your baby is hungry is by responding to their feeding cues. Early signs of hunger include stirring, turning their head or opening their mouth. As your baby's movement increases and they begin to stretch, they are starting to get hungrier. If they are agitated or crying, they're very hungry.

Breastfeeding

Breastmilk helps build your baby's immune system to protect them from illness and infection, and its nutritional benefits are well established. It's also full of hundreds of flavours from the mother's diet, which helps develop your child's tastebuds. In fact, breastfeeding is one of the best ways to influence your child's eating habits because they can taste what you are eating.

For mothers, the first six months post-delivery can take an incredible toll on your body, particularly if you're breastfeeding your newborn baby. You'll likely experience fatigue and exhaustion – and a noticeable increase in appetite. Making breastmilk is hard work for your body; it burns a lot of calories! After all, you're feeding another person. Try to keep this front of mind every time you worry about how hungry you are. It's a good thing that your appetite is increasing and a sign your body is working efficiently, for you and your baby. You need to listen to your body and give it the nutrition it needs.

While breastfeeding, what you feed yourself is just as important as what you feed your child. Don't be concerned about the volume of food you are eating; in fact, you must be diligent with your food intake and don't skip any meals, because this will only result in cravings for less healthy foods. Remember to eat the full rainbow, and stick to wholesome, nutritious foods, saving processed and fast food for a once-a-week treat. As you wean your baby off breast-milk, you will find that your own appetite decreases.

Learning how to breastfeed your baby can be challenging, and it might take several months to build your confidence. If you are experiencing difficulties breastfeeding your baby, don't be scared to seek help. Advice can be sought from the Australian Breastfeeding Association (breastfeeding.asn.au) or the breastfeeding association relevant to your country. But if breastfeeding doesn't work for you and your baby, don't worry. There is a perfectly suitable alternative in formula milk.

Formula

For many, breastfeeding isn't possible or practical. All kids (and mothers) are different. Baby formula is the only safe alternative to breastmilk and is packed with the added vitamins, minerals and fats that babies need. No particular brand of formula is better for your baby than another; they all offer a similar nutritional value and quality. You do not need to give your child formula that is marketed higher in protein, either – the regular kind is just fine. In fact, research has indicated that higher protein formulas can have a detrimental effect on a baby's weight later in childhood, and they are harder to digest for newborns. And please do not, as some social media influencers suggest, make your own baby formula. It's never going to strike the right balance of nutrition that your child needs.

It's also important to stick to one kind of formula; if you change regularly between different brands, your baby might become fussy and not want to feed due to the difference in taste. It can also wreak havoc on your child's tummy as it tries to adjust to the new formula, leading to pain and excessive crying. If you have no choice but to switch – due to an intolerance or supply issue, for example – try to do it gradually by slowly weaning them off the old formula while gradually introducing the new formula. A good rule of thumb is to introduce one bottle of new formula per day, at the morning feed. Continue to increase the number of new-formula feeds over the course of four or five days until the switch is complete. Remember not to mix different formulas in the same bottle as it can result in unpleasant tummy issues for your child.

Unless your child has a specific intolerance or allergy, it's best to buy formula made from cow's milk, which the majority are. If you suspect your baby has an intolerance or allergy, check in with your healthcare professional as they might advise a different formula, such as a lactose-free, low-lactose or soy alternative. All of these types of formula are perfectly safe for your baby, but you should only use them as recommended by a healthcare professional and under medical supervision.

Breastmilk or formula is not needed after the age of 12 months.

Introducing solids

When your child turns six months old, it's time to start introducing a variety of solid foods into their diet while continuing to feed them breastmilk or formula. If they're expressing interest in the food you eat, and if they're developmentally ready to do so – for example, if they're able to sit up – you can start introducing tiny quantities of soft foods from four months of age. While breastmilk or formula should remain your child's main food source for at least 12 months, it's important to introduce solids by the age of six months, because that's when your child's nutritional requirements change: their iron, calcium and energy needs increase, and breastmilk or formula alone are no longer sufficient. Solid foods will provide the additional energy they need for their growth and development, and to help their bones, muscles and organs mature. Delaying solids beyond six months can increase your child's risk of nutrient deficiencies and food allergies, hinder their growth and development, and lead to fussy eating behaviours. The introduction of solid foods is also crucial to your child's learning and development, including their speech progress. Learning how to eat helps develop their speech because the muscles used in eating are the same muscles that, combined with voice, are used to produce sound.

There is no right or wrong choice as to what foods to introduce first or how to introduce them. But a good starting point is focusing on foods that are rich in iron, such as cooked pureed meat. It will involve trial and error, and it does require persistence to get your child on board. You might have to offer them a new food up to seven times before they'll try it. It's also very common for your child to love a particular food one day, then hate it the next.

Practice makes perfect, so let your child play with lots of foods and different textures in the first 12 months. It will be a messy process along the way – most of the food will end up on their face or on the floor. But this is all part of the art of learning how to eat. If you are lucky enough to have a garden or green space nearby, take the highchair outside in summer, sit on the grass or stick your child in the pram – then give it a hose down later.

Modifying foods to suit your child's needs

Introducing your child to solids doesn't need to be complicated, and it doesn't mean you need to cook them separate meals to the rest of the family. However, as you start to introduce solids, it's important to modify the foods to avoid your child choking. They can eat the same food as you; you'll just need to modify the consistency of their food because they can't chew yet. But, as time-poor parents juggling the demands of modern life, make it easy for yourself and stick to foods that can be easily adapted. For example, make a family meal using mince instead of steak. It's also best to start with single-ingredient foods that are easy for your child to digest, such as banana, avocado, sweet potato and carrot, before moving on to multi-ingredient meals as they get older. From 6 to 8 months your child will need their solid food to be finely mashed or pureed; from 8 to 12 months, their food should be mashed, chopped or cut up as finger food; and from 12 months on they can enjoy exactly the same food that you put on your plate.

In terms of quantity, your child's first meals may consist of just a teaspoon or two of solid food. But once they get the hang of eating, that amount will start to increase. As a general guide, start by giving your child a couple of teaspoons of solid food with two meals a day, and gradually increase the amount and variety of solids. By the time your child is nine months old, you can feed them up to one cup of solids at each main meal, while still giving them formula or breastmilk in between (about four times per day). At 12 months old, your child can eat three small meals a day, with healthy snacks in between, and cow's milk can replace breastmilk or formula. Many mothers continue breastfeeding beyond the 12-month mark, which is perfectly fine, as long as you include a wide selection of solid foods to prevent nutritional deficiencies that may stunt your child's growth and development.

These sample feeding schedules will help you visualise how solids can fit into your child's daily meals, as well as how much you can expect them to be eating at a particular age. But these schedules and amounts are just a rough guide. Tablespoon and cup sizes vary by region and country, and every child is different. The most important thing is to pay attention to your child's communication signs. As we discovered in chapter 2, forcing your child to eat when they're not interested isn't fun for either of you, and, over time, you will dampen their appetite regulation system, making it harder for your child to tune in to their body's natural hunger and fullness cues.

Child's age	Breast milk or formula	Solid food
4 to 6 months	700 to 1000 ml per day (5 to 8 feeds)	1 to 2 solid meals per day, consisting of: 1 to 4 tablespoons of cereal (1 to 2 times per day) *and* 1 to 4 tablespoons of fruit and vegetables (1 to 2 times per day)
6 to 8 months	700 to 1000 ml per day (4 to 6 feeds)	2 to 3 solid meals per day, consisting of: 1 to 3 tablespoons protein food, for example, meat, eggs or legumes (2 to 3 times per day) *and* 4 to 9 tablespoons cereal, fruit and vegetables (2 to 3 times per day)
9 to 12 months	450 to 850 ml per day (3 to 5 feeds)	3 solid meals per day, consisting of: ¼ to ½ cup grain foods (2 times per day) *and* ¼ to ½ cup fruit (2 times per day) *and* ¼ to ½ cup vegetables (2 times per day) *and* ¼ cup dairy foods (2 times per day) *and* ¼ cup protein foods (2 times per day)

Baby-led weaning versus purees

How to start giving your child solids is often presented as a choice between 'baby-led weaning' – where you allow them to try your food, if it's in an appropriate form and consistency – and purees, where you give them foods that have been blended into a smooth puree. Many of you will be familiar with the scene of the parent delivering pureed or mashed food on a baby spoon into a child's wide-open mouth, with all the accompanying aeroplane sound effects. This is what we call conventional spoon-feeding. But for parents and caregivers who use baby-led weaning, the child's mealtime looks very different. Baby-led weaning involves letting your child self-feed with appropriate finger food instead, such as bite-sized pieces of fish or meat, steamed veggies, chopped fruit, sliced cheese or cooked wholemeal pasta

There are pros and cons to each method. Research shows that conventional spoon-feeding results in your child consuming more of the food, meaning they're more likely to meet their nutritional requirements, particularly when it comes to nutrients they won't get from milk, such as iron, which becomes more important from six months of age. On the other hand, baby-led weaning fine-tunes their motor development, including hand-eye coordination and chewing skills. It also helps them learn to self-regulate their appetite, and, more importantly, it prevents us as parents from disturbing this in-built self-regulation by forcing them to eat when they might not be hungry. Children who self-feed do not eat more than they need, since they are consuming their food independently. But when conventional spoon-feeding is used, parents often sneak a couple of extra mouthfuls of food into their baby's mouth, even if the baby is turning their head away and signalling that they are full.

When it comes to introducing your child to solids, the best approach is a mixture of both. Baby-led weaning is great for when you're having dinner as a family, because your child can eat little bits of appropriate food that the whole family is eating, instead of having a separate meal or needing to be spoon-fed. But if you're out and about, taking little jars of pureed baby food to spoon-feed your child can be convenient and time saving. This is the best way of ensuring they meet their nutritional needs while also developing those essential motor skills. You also don't need to stick to a rigorous schedule of breakfast, lunch and dinner – instead, try feeding your child solids when they are hungry and when it is convenient for you.

All supermarkets sell a range of baby purees, some of which are better than others in terms of ingredients. For time-poor parents, there are plenty of suitable options. You want to buy the ones with the fewest possible ingredients and that include only natural sources, such as apple, pear and oats, rather than purees that contain extenders or acids – which are perfectly safe to consume but do not provide your child with any nutritional benefits. If you can recognise all the ingredients on the list, and it doesn't include added sugar or salt, it's a great pick. It's also a good idea to stay clear of food pouches that have water as the first ingredient as it means you won't be getting much of the other ingredients in the puree, such as meat or veggies. Make sure the puree you choose is age appropriate – some are fine to feed your child from the age of four or six months; others are for when they are a little older. Of course, you can also puree whatever you're eating at home in the blender too.

'Food before one is just for fun'
This saying has certainly gained popularity in recent years, but there is no evidence to this claim – it's simply a catchy rhyme. There is no doubt about the importance of

continuing to feed your child breastmilk or formula beyond the age of six months. In fact, breastmilk or formula should be your child's main source of nutrition until they are 12 months old. But this doesn't mean food before one is just for fun: introducing your four- to six-month-old to solid foods is vital to provide your baby with the nutrients and energy they need to grow and thrive, as well as many developmental and social benefits, that cannot be obtained from breastmilk or formula alone.

What should you feed your child?

The answer is simple: whole foods. They're the most satisfying of all foods, and they're the most nutritious too! When foods are tested in the laboratory, they are ascribed a value that scientists refer to as the satiety index. Refined foods, such as white bread, chips, cake, croissants and other baked goods, are low in satiety and not as filling, meaning we often eat more of them than is good for us. On the other hand, whole foods are high on the satiety index and fill us up for long periods of time. These include fresh fruit and vegetables, whole grains, beans, nuts and meat – foods found in their natural state and typically high in fibre and protein, keeping you fuller for longer while also giving you the nutrients and energy needed to thrive. Filling your child up on wholesome and nutritious foods will help displace less healthy choices in their diet.

The simplest way to know what to feed your child is to learn what foods can be eaten every day and what foods should only be eaten sometimes. This distinction might be helpful for you to remember when deciding what to eat yourself, too! Bearing this in mind, the basis of your child's daily food intake should include the following everyday foods:

- Unlimited fruit and vegetables (all are suitable but let them enjoy a variety). Despite what you may have heard, your child can never eat too much fruit and veg. It's also perfectly fine if your child eats a lot of fruit and very little veg – they're still getting the necessary nutrition for healthy growth and development.
- Plenty of full-fat dairy products such as milk, cheese, cream cheese and yoghurt, or suitable dairy-free alternative foods in the case of allergies. You can give your child cow's milk with breakfast, lunch and dinner up to the age of two, and with breakfast and dinner from then on.
- Lots of 100 per cent nut butter of any kind is fine from the age of six months, or nuts (two large tablespoons or a large handful per day, as a guide) when they are at least five years old (to avoid choking).
- A wholegrain carbohydrate with three meals per day. For example, wholegrain bread or pasta, brown rice or other coloured rice, barley, buckwheat, oats or quinoa.
- Plenty of fish or seafood with at least three meals per week. You can try boneless fish fillets, tinned tuna or prawns. If your child has allergies, the omega-3 they'd typically get from eating seafood can instead be sourced from foods like nuts and seeds, canola oil or fortified foods like eggs.
- Protein – lean or 'heart smart' cuts of meat (be sure to trim all visible forms of fat off the meat), tofu, legumes or eggs – with each of the three main meals per day.
- Water, with all snacks and meals.

While whole foods can be eaten every day, 'sometimes' foods should only be eaten occasionally by you and your child – ideally once per week, and no more than twice per week. Similarly, fast food, takeaway or dining out should also be kept to once or twice per week for the whole family.

The following foods are just a few examples, not an exhaustive list, of what should be kept in the 'sometimes' basket. These 'sometimes' foods include: chips; biscuits; snack bars, energy bars or muesli bars; lollies and chocolate; savoury baked goods and pastries; ice cream; and cakes (including banana bread – don't let the fruit in the name fool you!). The main reason for these foods being on the 'sometimes' list is because they are very low in nutrition (or have no nutrition) and/or are packed full of 'empty calories' – calories that don't provide nutrition and won't fill you or your child up.

A good rule of thumb is to think of anything processed or found in the confectionary aisle as a 'sometimes' food. Clever marketing and misleading food packaging can make things confusing, so be mindful that just because something is labelled 'health food', 'gluten free', 'dairy free', 'wheat free' or 'vegan' doesn't mean it is better for your child. It might still be loaded with added sugar and fat and needs to be thought of as an occasional treat, not an everyday food. You might find it helpful to let your child choose their favourite treat, so they have control over what they're eating.

The importance of grocery shopping

Grocery shopping is not easy, and doing it with little ones is even harder. But even though it requires time and effort, shopping for your family is always going to be more satisfying and healthier and will save you a ton of money when compared to eating pre-packaged meals or takeaway food, and it should be your first choice.

To limit you and your child's exposure to 'sometimes' foods, your grocery shopping should be done once a week or so to make sure there is always plenty of healthy everyday food at home.

You could also consider ordering your family's groceries online and having it delivered, if you're in a position to do so. The weekly food shop will not change much from week to week, which makes ordering online even easier as your foods will be saved from the previous week's purchase. It might save you time and stress as you won't run the risk of your kid having a tantrum in the store or nagging you during the whole shop to buy them junk. Plus, the extra time you've saved from that risky shopping expedition can be devoted to a more fun and fulfilling activity, like playing with the kids at the park.

But rest assured, if you do your grocery shopping in person, there are many benefits to be gained from taking your child with you. They want to be involved in everything you do, so if it's not going to cause you too much angst, take them shopping too. Just make sure you have a contingency plan in case they throw a tantrum, because the supermarket – surrounded by unlimited food choices – is an environment where it's likely to happen. Children often act out because of hunger, tiredness and boredom, so be sure to feed your child beforehand and ensure they are well rested before hitting the supermarket.

If you're going to the shops, it's important to take a list with you so you don't forget anything (an example list is included later in this chapter). If your children are old enough, try involving them in the shopping process by asking them to find certain items for you or teaching them how to find the best value for money by comparing the price per 100 grams or 100 ml for different brands of the same food. For younger kids, sitting in the trolley watching you pick healthy options while ignoring the packaged stuff is also a valuable lesson.

You could also break up your grocery shopping into categories by taking your child with you to buy fruit and vegetables from your local fruit shop and meat from your local butcher, and then grabbing staples from one of the supermarket chains by yourself.

After all, supermarkets are where the problems arise when shopping with kids. They are designed to guide us around the perimeter of the store and to make trips up and down every aisle. It is unsurprising that products located at the end of the aisles and at checkout counter displays account for nearly half of all sales of packaged sweets. They are stacked with soft drinks, sweets, chips and baked goods rather than the fresh whole foods that are best for the health of you and your child.

Shopping list

Before you go grocery shopping for the week, it is a good idea to meal plan. Meal planning will also make it easier to write a list for your shopping trip. If your child is old enough, get them involved in the process too – try flicking through some recipe books together for inspiration, or pick your favourite recipes online. Not only does meal planning save you time, but it will save you money by preventing impulse buys during the week and it will prepare your children for what's to come that week.

You can use the following list to form the basis of your grocery shopping going forward. Keep a good supply of these foods and staples in your kitchen and when you start running low, make sure you add them to your shopping list before they run out. This list can be tailored based on some of your family's preferences or eating practices, such as vegetarianism. The most important thing to bear in mind is that each meal you cook should include plenty of salad or vegetables, as well as a wholegrain carbohydrate, a source of protein and a source of fat.

I know this list might seem overwhelming at first, but many of the items on it are staples that will last you a long time. If you're new to cooking, these ingredients can be accumulated gradually, as you and your family's confidence and skills develop.

Condiments, sauces and pastes: balsamic vinegar; honey; minced garlic, ginger and chilli (all natural, jarred with vinegar only); lemon juice (bottled); vegetable, chicken and beef stock (salt-reduced cubes or liquid in cartons); soy sauce; tomato paste (low salt); and 100 per cent nut butter.

Dried goods: baking powder; breadcrumbs; couscous; noodles; pulses (lentils, chickpeas, black beans, split peas); rice (basmati, brown, arborio); sugar; unsalted, dry-roasted or raw nuts; a variety of seeds (sunflower, flaxseed, pepitas, sesame); pasta; rolled oats; and wholemeal flour (plain and self-raising).

Dried herbs, seasoning and spices: basil; black pepper; salt; chilli flakes; parsley; thyme; rosemary; paprika; oregano; nutmeg; turmeric; cumin; and cinnamon.

Fresh fruits and vegetables: all types, and depending on your meal plans for the week.

Frozen goods: berries; edamame beans; filo pastry; and frozen vegetables (all varieties).

Long-lasting vegetables: garlic; ginger; onions; potato, regular and sweet; and pumpkin.

Oils: olive or canola oil (liquid can be decanted into a spray bottle).

Perishables: eggs; milk; yoghurt; wholegrain bread; fish; and meat.

Tinned or jarred food: beetroot; beans; capers; corn; chickpeas; fish (tuna or salmon in spring water or olive oil); lentils; olives; pineapple; and tomatoes. In our household we tend to buy tinned chickpeas and lentils as they are more convenient but if you have time, go for the dried option.

Food is expensive and grocery shopping is time-consuming, so don't worry or feel bad if you can't swing this whole list in one go. It is a guide only, and one that you can use to stock your fridge and pantry over time. The most important thing is focusing on making healthy and easy meals for you and your child.

To elaborate on the foods included on this shopping list and the food you should be giving your child – and the whole family – it's best to break them up into categories: fruits and vegetables; wholegrain carbs; lean protein sources; healthy fats; dairy; snacks and spreads; condiments; fermented foods; tinned and frozen foods; and beverages and treats.

Fruits and vegetables

There are *no* bad fruits or vegetables. Despite what you may have been told, bananas and potatoes won't make you or your child overweight, and they won't raise your blood sugar level or worsen your risk of developing type 2 diabetes. In fact, they reduce it. All fruits and vegetables – including bananas and potatoes – are packed with vitamins, minerals and fibre (both soluble and insoluble fibre, and resistant starch) and are good for you and your child's health.

Insoluble fibre is found in the skin of fruits and vegetables, and it ensures you have regular bowel movements. Soluble fibre is found in the flesh of fruits and vegetables, and it helps keep cholesterol levels in the healthy range by mopping up 'bad' cholesterol (LDL cholesterol, which can increase your risk of stroke and heart disease) and removing it from your blood. And those potatoes that you might worry about giving your child? Well, they are high in resistant starch. The trick is to first bake them and then allow them to cool; that way they are packed with resistant starch, another type of fibre that has a prebiotic effect, meaning it promotes plenty of good bacteria and microbes in the gut. Of course, there are plenty of other great sources of these three types of fibre, such as wholegrain breads and cereals, pasta, nuts and seeds, lentils, peas and beans, but it's good to remember that 'sometimes' foods we fear are actually the ones we need plenty of for our overall well-being. Without them, you could be putting your kid's health at risk, and it may not even be evident for many years down the track.

Fruit and vegetables do contain sugars, but they are naturally occurring sugars, which are also not bad for your child's health. In fact, research has proven that they help prevent heart disease, type 2 diabetes and cancer, meaning a whole range of fresh fruit and veg – the full rainbow – should be part of your family's daily eating plan. You don't need to limit how much fruit your child eats, even if they eat way more fruit than veg. Sweeter vegetables, such as peas, corn, pumpkin and sweet potato, are more likely to be accepted than bitter vegetables such as broccoli and cauliflower. I'm not saying don't offer a wide variety of options for your child to try, but I do recommend focusing on regularly including what you know they will eat. Roasting veggies such as pumpkin and sweet potato in the oven also brings out their natural sweetness, increasing the likelihood that your child will eat them. And don't bother putting bitter vegetables such as cauliflower or broccoli by themselves on the plate; your child won't go anywhere near them. Yes, it's important to encourage children to enjoy vegetables for their texture as well as their taste, but this is something they're more likely to embrace as they get older, during their schooling years. Try sneaking those bitter veggies on a pizza, roasted, or include them in bolognaise, sauces, soups and casseroles by cooking and then blitzing them up. These 'hidden' veggies are a good way to get vegetables your child doesn't like into their diet. For example, spaghetti can include blitzed-up broccoli, lentils and tomatoes, while homemade burger patties can include grated carrot and corn kernels.

Much of the confusion around foods containing sugar (such as fruits) originates from the sugar-free message promoted by diet companies. Advocates for sugar-free diets suggest avoiding table sugar, some natural sweeteners like maple syrup and honey, sweets, condiments, soft drinks and a selection of fruits – an arbitrary list of foods to avoid, which has no substance to its claim of being good for your health. Many of the foods that are blacklisted, such as honey and berries, contain naturally occurring sugars, which, as we now know, help prevent a whole range of health concerns. This sort of messaging is not based on scientific evidence. Many of the sugar-free recipes that diet companies promote still contain sugar, but they are cleverly disguised as expensive sugar alternatives, such as rice malt syrup, and often the same companies that flog sugar-free diets or programs also sell these ingredients. Pushing any sort of restrictive diet, including a sugar-free diet, onto your child will do more harm than good, and it may result in them obsessing about their eating habits as they grow up, living in fear that they will eat something that's not allowed or 'bad'. Instead of promoting a dieting mentality and obsession with weight loss and body image in the family household – inadvertently or not – try encouraging your child to eat the full rainbow, and model this behaviour for them yourself.

The sugar conundrum

There is no debating that we need to reduce our kids' consumption of sugar, but this needs to happen by reducing our intake of processed foods like sweets, muesli bars, baked goods, soft drinks, cakes and chocolate – all of which contain added or refined sugars. When it comes to packaged foods, sugar wears many different disguises. Recent research shows that added sugars hide behind more than 40 different names in the ingredients lists, so that's why it's more important to focus on reducing the consumption of these packaged foods rather than pondering a bunch of items at the supermarket all day looking for healthier alternatives. Instead, try giving your child a piece of fruit containing naturally occurring sugars. You don't need to limit the amount of fruit they're eating – having more than two pieces of fruit per day is not going to harm them. In fact, it's going to do the exact opposite; it will make them healthier.

Wholegrain carbs

Wholegrain carbohydrates are another great source of nutrition; they're packed with vitamins and minerals and are a rich source of fibre. Focus on including one source of wholegrain carbohydrate with every family meal. This is easy if you start early, when you first start introducing your child to solids, but if they're already a little older, it's a bit more challenging. We acquire certain tastes and food preferences from a very early age, so if your child is used to a lifetime of white bread and white pasta, you might be met with some resistance when you make the switch to wholegrain versions. Patience is key! Try introducing these foods gradually, with your child's involvement. It also helps to explain why you're making the switch and how these foods are better for the whole family. If your child feels in control, it increases the likelihood of them eating it.

Whole grains, or foods made with them, contain all components of the original wheat kernel (the bran, germ and endosperm). All of these must be present for something to qualify as a wholegrain food. Foods such as couscous, white bread, white pasta and white rice do not contain whole grains. That's not to say your child can't eat them; they just shouldn't be as prevalent in their diet as their wholegrain cousins. For some items, such as bread and pasta, you might need to check the packaging or ingredients list to make sure you are buying a wholegrain version, but other forms of whole grains, such as amaranth, buckwheat, bulgur, freekeh and oats, are invariably wholegrain versions.

Whole grains include: wholegrain or dark rye bread; wholegrain pasta; brown, black, purple or red rice; whole or hulled barley (avoid pearled, as that means it has been processed and some or all of the bran has been removed); buckwheat; bulgur; whole corn, rye, spelt, wheat and farro or emmer (again, avoid pearled); freekeh; millet; oats (steel-cut or rolled oats are preferred but refined or 'quick' oats are more suitable for infants less than two years of age); quinoa; and wild rice. Many of these exotic grains might sound intimidating and like something a child would never eat; if you are looking at those names in disbelief, I suggest starting with a bowl of porridge for brekkie! If you get your child hooked on the nutritious stuff from an early age, they will never know any different and won't be crying out for the packaged cereal or white bread when you go grocery shopping.

Breads

Bread is a dietary staple in many households, and with good reason; it's nutritious and filling, as long as you opt for the healthier, wholegrain options. Better still, sandwiches make for a very easy and convenient lunch option for children, particularly if you're on the go or short on time. But with all the different bread choices available nowadays, it can be quite overwhelming to know what you should and shouldn't be buying. As you ponder the supermarket shelves, you'll find wholegrain, multigrain, wholemeal, sourdough, rye, white, high-fibre white, low glycaemic index (low GI) and gluten-free options, and often a plethora of different brands for each type.

White bread is refined as the wheat kernels it contains have had the bran and germ removed. Its nutritional value is low, and it's not something you should be feeding your child every day. It won't fill them up for long periods and they'll be more likely to overeat.

Wholemeal bread is made from whole grains that have been milled to a fine texture, which gives it a plain brown appearance. It's a step up from white bread, containing more nutrition and making it the sensible choice for children less than two years of age as it doesn't pose any potential choking hazards that can be associated with grainy breads.

Multigrain bread is often confused with wholegrain bread, but there is a difference. Multigrain is made from white flour with whole grains added back in. It's a better and more nutritious option than white or wholemeal bread, but it's not as healthy as a true wholegrain version.

Wholegrain bread contains the entire grain or wheat kernel – the bran (outer layer), endosperm (starchy middle layer) and germ (nutrient-rich inner part). It has a dense wholemeal flour base with grains and seeds. Soy and linseed bread are a variety of wholegrain bread with added healthy omega-3 fatty acids, a form of essential fat that is good for our brain health.

Then there's rye and sourdough bread. Wholegrain rye bread is the best of the rye options, but light rye is still better than white bread. The same applies for sourdough – a wholegrain sourdough is the best choice of all the sourdough breads. Authentic sourdough (made without yeast and utilising another starter instead) can be quite expensive as it takes a long time to produce and results in an acidic, quite chewy or tough bread. Sourdough is best avoided for young children; they can find it very hard to eat due to its texture.

When it comes to gluten-free breads, they are made with alternative grains to wheat, to avoid the wheat protein: gluten. If your child is diagnosed with coeliac disease, gluten-free options are a suitable alternative to wholegrain bread (more on this in the next section). But if your child is not coeliac or otherwise diagnosed as gluten-intolerant, there's no need to be buying this more expensive alternative as they're not healthier than regular breads. It is important to include a type of bread your child can tolerate, especially as bread is a good source of folate – another one of those vitamins that your child needs to grow and thrive.

The general rule of thumb is to buy wholemeal bread for children less than two years of age, and multigrain or wholegrain bread for children over two years of age. Even though they are more processed, the occasional wholemeal or wholegrain pita bread is also not going to hurt your child (we love making wraps in our household). Just make sure that the words 'wholemeal', 'whole-wheat' or 'whole-wheat flour' is the first ingredient on the label and that 'wholegrain' is high in the ingredient list. Generally speaking, the darker the bread looks, the better it's going to be for your child. My tip is to keep bread in the freezer so you can get out what you want when you need it.

When it comes to selecting the best brand, they're all pretty similar, especially the commercial varieties found in the supermarket. It is now a legal requirement that all bread-making flour contains folate (vitamin B-9) and iodised salt (for thyroid health), but organic breads are exempt from this legalisation. Folate is not just important for growing children, it's vital during pregnancy too as it's needed for the growth and formation of your little one's neural tube in the first few weeks after conception. The neural tube forms the brain and spinal cord, and without enough folate the tube won't fuse properly and could cause a neural tube defect, such as spina bifida. Iodine (i.e. iodised salt) is also needed for the development of your child's brain and nervous system. So when it comes to buying bread for your growing child, commercial varieties are typically the better option.

Bread and gluten

Coeliac disease is an autoimmune disorder triggered by the consumption of gluten, a protein found in wheat, rye and barley that gives products like bread their elasticity and texture. This disease affects 1 per cent of the world population (1 in 70 Australians). When people with coeliac disease eat gluten, it damages their small intestine meaning they can't absorb nutrients from food. They end up with unpleasant side effects, such as itchy skin, heartburn, diarrhoea, bloating and constipation. Gluten is not dangerous for the rest of the population, and it doesn't cause cancer. In fact, cutting it out of your diet unnecessarily can do more harm than good. Research has proven that a diet rich in wholegrain carbs and fibre – such as breads and cereals – will reduce, not increase, your child's risk of developing colon cancer.

Despite this evidence, the number of people following a 'gluten-free' diet has tripled in the past 10 years and it all starts in the family household. Many parents who go on, or put their child on, a gluten-free diet have not been diagnosed with coeliac disease, and if they've experienced similar symptoms, it could well be due to something entirely different to a gluten intolerance. Other parents cut out gluten because they think it's fattening. Every gram of carbohydrate – which is stored as glycogen in the body – binds three times its weight in water. Put simply, eating carbs (and the gluten it contains) can make the number on the scale go up. Cutting carbs or gluten might make that number go down, only it isn't a decrease in fat mass, but rather a decrease in water content in the body. If you start eating more processed food to compensate for cutting out healthy wholegrain carbs, instead choosing gluten-free biscuits, crackers or other packaged goods, it's not a healthier choice. Many of these products are higher in fat, salt and sugar, and lower in protein and fibre, than their regular counterparts in order to make them more palatable.

The only way to determine whether you or your child has coeliac disease is to get tested by your doctor. They may suggest a blood test in the first instance, but the gold standard test is an endoscopy, where a gastroenterologist will stick a tube with a camera on it down your or your child's throat to examine the lining of the intestine. Pretty intense stuff. Even if you or your child don't have coeliac disease, you may still have an intolerance to gluten, causing you to have an upset stomach when you eat it. In this instance, gluten-free breads may be a better option for your family. But it's also important to eat suitable whole grains that are naturally gluten-free and also rich in fibre, such as rice and quinoa, rather than eating only white gluten-free bread, in order to derive the benefits of whole grains.

Pasta

Wholegrain pasta is always the preferred option as it's higher in fibre than regular or white pasta. Chickpea pasta is also a great one to add to the rotation. But any pasta is fine in moderation; the focus of any pasta dish needs to be meal balance. Pasta should be eaten the Mediterranean way – that is, with an accompanying salad, so that half of the meal is the pasta and meat, and the other half is the salad. For small children, try giving them baked vegetables, such as pumpkin and sweet potato, instead of salad. They're more likely to go for them due to their natural sweetness.

Cereals

Cereals are a breakfast staple in many households, and understandably so – they're quick and easy, and kids tend to love them. But instead of sugary, processed and packaged cereals, stick to oats, natural muesli and any wholegrain-based cereals, such as Weet-Bix or All-Bran. The other cereals can be left on the supermarket shelves, otherwise your kid will be starving by 9 a.m.

Rice

The healthier options are brown rice and, if it's within your budget, red or black rice. But much like all wholegrain foods, these types of rice taste very different from their white counterparts and, consequently, can be challenging to introduce to your child later in life. Don't be shocked if they scrunch their nose at you when you first give it to them! Just keep trying. Basmati rice is also a decent option and better suited to some dishes, particularly Asian cuisine. Black rice and red rice are delicious, but they're often two to three times the price of brown rice and they don't suit all dishes. You can also consider alternative grains such as quinoa or barley – but don't feel you have to include them, if you can't find them or can't afford them. White rice is not the best of the rice varieties, but it's still better than a drive-through or takeaway meal!

Lean protein sources

We all need protein, but too much of it can be detrimental to your child's health. You should include a source of lean protein with each family meal, but the entire meal shouldn't be made up of protein.

There are plenty of protein sources that are suitable for your child. Chicken breasts or thighs, 'heart smart' or lean mince, lamb cutlets or sizzle steak are all fine for children. Chicken drumsticks are also suitable. It is easy to pick out the leanest cuts of meat as they will have less marbling or white fatty tissue visible; the white part is the fat. If your child isn't eating meat, include plenty of fish, legumes (including lentils), eggs and tofu in your family's meals. These are all healthy alternatives to meat that are also rich sources of nutrition and protein.

Cheaper cuts of meat – blade or porterhouse steaks – from cattle tend to be the toughest and are best for slow-cooked dishes where the protein breaks down over time to give the meat its tenderness.

Slow-cooked dishes make it easy to feed the whole family and can bubble away safely in a slow cooker while you do other things. Add some meat, stock and chopped veggies to the slow cooker pot in the morning and allow it to stew while you do a day's work. These cheaper cuts of meat are perfectly fine from a nutritional point of view and make a difference only to your wallet and method of cooking.

Lamb is a great alternative to beef and packed full of flavour, but unless you can afford the premium cuts, it is a much fattier meat, so limit the lamb chops to just once per fortnight. Lamb cutlets, on the other hand, can be enjoyed regularly. Save all varieties of pork to a maximum of once per week, particularly the processed forms, such as bacon and ham, because pork is a much fattier meat alternative to beef and lamb. Lastly, keep processed meats – sliced meats, chorizo or salami – to the 'treat' or 'sometimes' food category as they are preserved with additives and extra salt to prolong their shelf life.

Meat myths

There is no reason why every family meal needs to contain meat. Your child will get all their iron needs from three meals containing meat per week, and it's better to include a variety of protein-rich food sources in their diet rather than relying solely on meat. Try making some vegetarian meals where legumes, eggs or tofu are the source of protein; these foods are a nutritionally sound alternative to meet you and your child's protein needs.

Eggs

If you're wondering whether you need to limit the number of eggs you and your child eat, the answer is no! We were told for decades that dietary cholesterol is bad for us, and it was thought that the cholesterol found in eggs increased the cholesterol in our blood. But this isn't true. Cholesterol can be produced naturally by the liver and it performs several vital roles in the body, including producing new cells and hormones that help the body function properly. Therefore, if you don't get enough cholesterol in your diet, your body will produce cholesterol itself. Your body needs cholesterol to survive. But the reverse also applies: when you get enough cholesterol from your diet, such as by eating eggs, your liver produces less of it.

Eggs are nutritious and a great source of protein. They also contain micronutrients that are important for eye and heart health and healthy blood vessels. Eating them will *not* increase the level of bad cholesterol in the blood. They make for great snacks when boiled, or you can serve them poached, scrambled made with milk, or fried with some olive oil. You need to introduce cooked egg to your child early on (from the age of four to six months) as the outcomes in terms of allergies are far better than if you hold off until they're older.

Seafood

Fish is a great source of protein and healthy fat, particularly omega-3, an essential fat your child needs for healthy brain and eye development. The best source of omega-3 is fish, and by including adequate amounts in your own diet during pregnancy, you will lower the risk of your child being born too early or with a low birth weight and ensure they develop a healthy thyroid and good metabolism. Omega-3 is also found in plant sources such as nuts and seeds, but converting plant-sourced omega-3 to its usable form is an inefficient process in the body.

Your child should be eating fish or seafood with at least three meals per week. The same guideline applies during pregnancy.

While research shows that mercury levels should be kept to a minimum, particularly while you are pregnant, and for children up to the age of six years, we know getting enough omega-3 and iodine is more important than the possible risk of consuming too much mercury. The best way to mitigate any potential risk is to eat fish regularly but keep deep-sea predators such as shark – the fish used in most fish and chips meals at shops, pubs or restaurants – marlin and swordfish to about once a fortnight, with no other fish consumed that week. If you do happen to eat one of these deep-sea types, don't panic; it's still fine to eat them, just not every day. Fish ingest mercury from streams and oceans as they feed, so the bigger and older they are, the more mercury they will contain. Other top-of-the-food-chain predatory fish that should be limited to being eaten about once per week include kingfish, tuna, orange roughy (deep sea perch), catfish, king mackerel and barramundi. Tinned tuna is perfectly fine to eat during pregnancy and to give regularly to your child. It makes for a great lunch with some brown rice or wholegrain crackers and salad. Tinned tuna mostly contains smaller species of tuna (such as skipjack tuna), and the mercury content is negligible, so it's hard to consume too much of it. Recent data shows that you would have to eat around 12 tins (95 g per tin) of tuna per week before you hit the upper limit of mercury recommended during pregnancy or for children two to six years of age – and that limit doubles for the rest of the population.

All shellfish are nutritious, and you can include any type in your child's diet – even prawns. Much like eggs, despite your possible concerns about prawns containing cholesterol, shellfish won't increase the cholesterol level in your child's blood – unless you're giving them prawns covered in batter, like those you get from the fish shop.

Another common question when it comes to seafood is whether it's better to buy farmed or wild-caught fish. Let's take salmon as an example. Nowadays much of the salmon you can buy isn't caught in the wild (i.e. in oceans, rivers or lakes) but instead bred in fish farms. In fact, globally, approximately 50 per cent of salmon comes from fish farms. Farmed salmon has a completely different diet (processed fish feed) to wild salmon (various invertebrates). Nutritionally, yes, there are differences. Farmed varieties contain more saturated fat than wild-caught salmon, but the differences are too small to worry about. However, due to the high density of fish in fish farms, they are more susceptible to infection and disease than wild fish. To counter this problem, antibiotics are added to their fish feed, but this process is tightly regulated in developed countries, and not of concern when it comes to your or your child's health. If you can afford to buy wild-caught Atlantic salmon, then go for it, but farmed salmon is also perfectly fine and it's what you're more likely to find in Australia. It's also the salmon we eat in our household.

You might also be worried about microplastics (very small pieces of plastic that pollute the environment) in wild fish, and the potential harm this can have on your child's health from consuming them. Research suggests that microplastics are not absorbed in significant amounts by marine life, and so their potential to cause problems for your child's health is very low.

We could discuss the differences between farmed and wild-caught fish all day. But as is the case with everything relating to the advice in this book and what the research shows, you don't need to worry about the small stuff. Instead, focus on the overall health of your whole family and regularly include fish in your child's eating plan. Remember to offer a variety of fish too; don't eat the same type of fish all the time. You can include salmon in your family's diet on a weekly basis, but it shouldn't be the only type of fish you eat. At our place, we like tinned tuna, sardines (extremely good value and sustainable, although deboning them for a small child is very annoying), whole barramundi or snapper cooked on the barbecue, prawns, salmon, whiting and mussels. The benefits of eating fish far outweigh any potential negatives. Cooked fish also lends itself well to being pureed or chopped into chunks for small children. Just be careful of bones! And while fish fingers are not the best way to feed your child, often being overly processed with added fats and other ingredients, hence offering less nutritional benefit compared to fresh fish, the occasional bit of packaged, crumbed fish accompanied by vegetables is fine.

Healthy fats

Fat plays an important role in many processes within the human body. A well-balanced meal for you and your child needs to have a source of healthy fat. Fats to keep in the 'sometimes' food category, include artificial trans fats and saturated fats, like those found in many packaged or processed foods. But unsaturated fats and omega-3 fatty acids are what we call 'good' or 'healthy' fats and will give you energy, help fight heart disease and even lower your blood pressure. Great sources of healthy fat include avocado, extra virgin olive oil, 100 per cent nut butters, nuts and seeds. These are some of nature's best treats.

Oils

There is certainly no shortage of choice when it comes to cooking oils. Oils play an important role in our diet – we use them for baking, frying, dressing salads and making marinades. They are also a source of fat that is essential for the production of cells and hormones, as well as helping the body absorb nutrients. They come in two forms – solid (saturated fat) or liquid (unsaturated fat).

Let's kick it off with coconut oil, because I know you're dying to ask. This has been one of the best marketing scams of the 21st century – although it's a close race between coconut oil, alkaline water, goji berries and almond milk. Coconut oil – much like alkaline water, goji berries and almond milk – shouldn't be part of your child's diet. Coconut oil is about 80 per cent saturated fat, which is why it's solid at room temperature. Government nutrition guidelines tell us to avoid coconut oil because of its detrimental effect on heart health – it has been shown to raise our low-density lipoprotein (LDL) cholesterol, otherwise known as our 'bad' cholesterol, which blocks our arteries and causes heart attacks. There are better oils (containing unsaturated fat) that can improve our heart health, so you shouldn't be putting coconut oil – white gunk, as I like to call it – in your child's body. Replacing sources of saturated with unsaturated fat will improve your child's health.

Olive oil is also very popular and a key part of the Mediterranean eating plan. It is obtained from the fruit of olive trees. Whether it be 'extra virgin', 'virgin', 'pure', 'lite' or 'light', all varieties of olive oil tick the box when it comes to nutrition. The Australian olive oil industry has exceptionally high standards guaranteeing a fresh and best quality product, so it is often better to buy a local brand rather than an imported one. You really do get what you pay for when it comes to oil. Olive oil is predominantly made up of unsaturated fat, which reduces the 'bad' cholesterol in our blood. Better still, olive oil is largely made up of monounsaturated fat rather than polyunsaturated fat. Both are unsaturated and considered healthy fats. But the modern-day Western diet has meant that you and your child are likely getting too much of one specific type of polyunsaturated fat called omega-6, typically contained in other oils and processed foods such as cakes, baked goods, biscuits and takeaway meals. Too much omega-6 leads to inflammation. However, a diet rich in olive oil and fish will decrease inflammation in the body and improve your child's overall wellbeing.

Extra virgin olive oil is the highest quality olive oil you can buy as it is extracted from the first pressing of olives and has not been subjected to temperature during extraction. That's why you often see 'cold pressed' on the label. You can use extra virgin olive oil for everything when it comes to cooking, but the smoke point – the temperature at which oil goes rancid – varies between the different types of olive oil due to the way they have been processed. You should never let the oil smoke when cooking, so if you find yourself in that position, clean the pan, turn down the heat on the stove and start again. If you follow this rule, you really can use extra virgin olive oil for everything – as a dip for bread or a dressing for salads, in marinades, and when cooking or baking. It is best stored in a dark, cool place to preserve its quality, and be sure to use it within 12 months of the harvest date (stated on the bottle) as this will ensure its freshness is retained. Other varieties of olive oil are subjected to higher temperatures during the extraction process and therefore contain less antioxidants than extra virgin olive oil. Any olive oil labelled 'pure' has been refined and is not 'extra virgin', and bottles labelled 'lite' or 'light' olive oil are simply lighter in flavour, not fat as you may have been led to believe. These are all still fine choices.

Canola oil (also known as rapeseed oil) is another popular oil that comes from the seeds of the canola plant – the same plants that produce the small, yellow flowers you might see when driving around regional Australia in spring. Much like olive oil, canola is high in monounsaturated fat and makes up a large part of the Nordic diet – another diet, much like the Mediterranean diet, proven to reduce the risk of heart disease. Canola oil has a neutral flavour and high smoke point, making it suitable for baking and stir-frying. Its limiting factor is that it's often found in highly refined forms, so it won't pack nearly as many nutritional benefits as extra virgin olive oil. But you can also buy unrefined or 'cold pressed' canola oil, which contains more antioxidants than its refined counterparts. It's also cheaper than olive oil and the next-best option for your family when it comes to oil.

Sunflower and safflower oil have the same nutritional break-down and are high in omega-6 polyunsaturated fats. Even though polyunsaturated fats are good for us, most children eat too much of them in the modern-day Western diet. Sunflower and safflower oil are versatile when it comes to cooking due to their high smoke points and light taste, which is why they're commonly used for deep-frying, but they're not something you should be putting in your shopping trolley. Research has also shown that oils rich in polyunsaturated fats, like sunflower and safflower oil, produce toxic substances known as aldehydes when heated, which are detrimental to your child's health.

When it comes to vegetable oil, just because it has the word 'vegetable' in it doesn't make it a healthy choice for your family. In fact, vegetable oils fall towards the bottom of the list when it comes to what oil to choose. The highly processed and refined extraction of various seeds results in a flavourless and odourless oil that can be subjected to high temperatures. This makes vegetable oil suitable for deep-frying, but like many of the oils from which it is derived – sunflower, safflower, sesame, peanut, cottonseed, palm – it is high in omega-6 polyunsaturated fat and is best left on the supermarket shelf.

You could write an entire book on all the different oils available, so I won't be able to get into them all here. If I haven't mentioned a particular oil, don't use it. Stick to olive and canola as the oils of choice in your household – bottled or spray versions are both fine.

The best way to dispose of oil – whether that's used cooking oil or oil drained from a jar of semi-dried tomatoes or similar – is to create an oil jar under your sink. Tip the used oil into that jar and seal until next time. When the jar is full, throw it in the bin. Pouring used oil down your sink is not good for the plumbing and it's bad for the environment.

Dairy

Dairy is one of the most important food groups for kids because it's rich in calcium, which is needed for strong bones. The first two decades of life are critical to building enough calcium mineral deposits to form the hard, yet resilient, tissue that is healthy bone. Without these calcium mineral deposits, your child's bones will be brittle and weak, making them more prone to fractures. But dairy is not only a source of calcium, it's also a great source of protein. And even though it contains fat – mainly saturated – studies have shown that not all saturated fat is equal, and the kind you find in dairy is not detrimental to your or your child's health.

Children under two years of age should only have full-fat dairy. For children over two, dietary guidelines recommend that they consume reduced-fat dairy rather than regular or full-fat varieties. This is because we don't have any high-quality randomised controlled trials that directly compare the effects of full-fat versus low-fat dairy intake on body weight in children. These studies are needed to provide better quality evidence in this area. However, other studies have clearly documented that children with more dairy products of any kind – milk, yoghurt and cheese, full fat or otherwise – in their diet have better heart health and are better able to manage their weight as they grow older than those who don't. But it's important to note that these are association studies that examine groups of people over time, not controlled studies where you can accurately determine if one thing causes another.

When it comes to milk, you can switch your child to skim or low-fat milk at two years of age, but as I mentioned, there's no real need. To explain the difference, these products have the fat skimmed off the top, so the saturated fat percentage is halved in the case of low-fat milk (so you end up with a product that has approximately 2 per cent fat) or completely removed in the case of skim or no fat (so you end up with a product of less than 0.2 per cent fat). This seems like a good thing in theory as you're reducing your child's saturated fat intake which should improve their health. But, when it comes to saturated fat, it's much more complicated than this. The research shows that the types of saturated fat found in milk (and other dairy, like yoghurt and cheese) present a different effect on risk factors for heart disease – specifically, no detrimental effect or even an improvement – when compared to other food sources of saturated fat, such as sausages and cakes. Therefore, full fat is perfectly fine for your child's heart health, but so too is skim or low-fat milk, because it contains little to no saturated fat content.

So, if you'd rather give your child full-fat dairy as they grow up, this is fine. The most important thing is that you include dairy in your child's diet every day. Many parents worry about the added sugar content found in dairy products such as yoghurt. It's always good to be careful when it comes to added sugar. You can buy no-fat and low-fat yoghurt without added sugar, or you can opt for full-fat plain yoghurt and add your own sweetness by using fruit, or alternatively honey, which is okay for children from 12 months of age. Cheese is another healthy dairy product and makes for a great children's snack too.

Dairy intolerance and milk alternatives

Nowadays, there's a type of milk for every lifestyle, with countless milk options (just like bread and cooking oils) taking up nearly a whole aisle in the supermarket. Long gone are the days when the biggest decision was deciding between full-cream or low-fat milk. Instead, we wander the supermarket struggling to decide between soy milk, A2 milk, rice milk, oat milk, coconut milk, hemp milk and almond milk – not to mention all the other types of nut milk.

Whether it be full-cream, low-fat or skim milk, all varieties of cow's milk tick the box when it comes to nutrition. Cow's milk has significantly more protein than nut milks. It's also a rich source of calcium and vitamin D, also needed for healthy bones, and iodine, which helps ensure healthy thyroid function and weight control. The only difference between full-fat and skim milk is the energy content, as the fat has been stripped off the top, with skim varieties containing about half the calories of full-cream milk. However, not all children can tolerate cow's milk because it contains lactose, a naturally occurring sugar. Children who are unable to digest lactose (in fact, up to two-thirds of the global population struggle to absorb lactose) suffer from gastrointestinal side effects such as diarrhoea and bloating. They can still tolerate a splash of milk, but they can't enjoy a whole milkshake without some negative side effects. Lactose-free milk is a suitable option for those who are lactose intolerant as the lactase sugar has been removed from the milk, allowing them to enjoy the dairy product without any unpleasant symptoms. Nutritionally, it is the same as regular cow's milk, it tastes very similar, and it's readily available nowadays.

One of the biggest growing brands is A2 milk. Cow's milk contains both the A1 and A2 milk proteins. Some cows also produce only the A2 milk protein, which is the product you see on the supermarket shelves called A2 milk. There is no nutritional difference between the products, but A2 milk will cost you double the price. If you can afford it and prefer it, then great, but there is no health reason you need to be buying it for your child. The A1 milk protein is certainly not detrimental to your child's health, and it's likely that anyone who experiences fewer gastrointestinal side effects from drinking A2 milk will also experience the same benefits when drinking lactose-free milk.

This brings me to the extensive list of milk alternatives that are growing in popularity. Almond milk would have to be one of the most talked about food products in the 21st century, alongside coconut oil. Almond milk is made by grinding up almonds and adding water. It's a rich source of calcium but very low in protein. It's also expensive due to its high production cost, and it contains other ingredients such as stabilisers, emulsifiers and sometimes vegetable oils. Some brands will also be sweetened with added sugar. Almond milk, or any type of nut milk, is not an appropriate milk substitute for infant formulas, or for toddlers or older children. Almond milk is also bad for the environment because of the huge volume of water and number of bees required to cultivate the almonds used in it.

Other hugely popular milk alternatives include oat milk, coconut milk and rice milk. Oat milk is made from whole oats but will also contain other ingredients, such as sunflower oil. It's higher in carbohydrates than other milks and therefore will have a small fibre content, but milk is not a food we typically source our fibre from. With respect to its protein and calcium content, oat milk stacks up pretty well; it has half the protein of cow's milk, much higher than all the different types of nut milk, and the majority of brands will be calcium fortified. Like coconut oil, coconut milk is high in saturated fat, contains no protein and is very low in calcium. Coconut products are certainly very popular, but the evidence doesn't stack up when it comes to the benefits of including them in your or your child's diet. It also comes at a higher cost. Rice milk is another popular milk hitting our cafes and the supermarket shelves. It's made from whole brown rice and other ingredients, such as sunflower oil. As with nut milk, it's very low in protein and calcium. However, there are calcium-fortified varieties of rice milk on the supermarket shelves. But rice, oat or other alternative nut milks should never be provided as a replacement for breastmilk or formula for young children.

And then there's soy milk. Soy milk is a liquid extract of soybeans. Unlike all the other milk alternatives, this one gets a true tick of approval. It's a very popular cow's milk substitute – with good reason, as unlike all the other dairy alternatives, it matches regular milk for calcium and protein content. This is the best choice if your child can't tolerate cow's milk or the lactose-free variety. Just make sure to buy the 'calcium-fortified' or 'calcium-enriched' varieties and avoid soy milk that is low in calcium. The one thing lacking in soy when compared to cow's milk is iodine – which is needed to manage your child's weight – and large amounts of soy combined with an inadequate intake of iodine can also exacerbate iodine deficiency. But there are plenty of food sources rich in iodine, including seafood and commercial breads. Don't get caught up in the hype about soy being detrimental to your child's health or causing cancer; it's not true.

Snacks and spreads

The best snacks for your child are ones that are filling and nutritious. Suitable suggestions include wholemeal or wholegrain toast, or wholegrain crackers with cheese, avocado, jam (no added sugar) or 100 per cent nut butter (for example, peanut butter, cashew butter or almond butter). Peanut butter isn't fattening or bad for your child's health. They can have it every day, as long as you make sure to buy one that is made from 100 per cent peanuts and doesn't contain any added sugar or salt. The only thing on the ingredients label should be 100 per cent nuts.

Nuts are one of those foods that parents tend to stay away from because of the 'F' word: fat. We continue to cling onto the low-fat weight-loss message that came out in the 1980s – despite it since being dispelled – coupled with the low-fat marketing campaign that we still see proclaimed on the packaging of an abundance of products in supermarkets.

The truth is, nuts are high in fibre, protein, antioxidants, vitamins and minerals. They are also packed with good-for-you unsaturated fats. The good source of fat, fibre and protein found in nuts makes them a great snack for your child and will keep them fuller for longer. Not only do nuts make you feel fuller but they also speed up your metabolism as not all the calories from nuts are absorbed when they're eaten. In fact, 20 per cent of the energy from nuts is not absorbed at all, meaning they give you a feeling of fullness without causing weight gain.

You can give your child a couple of tablespoons of peanut butter, or any other variety of nut butter every day. This is just a guide and it's perfectly fine to give them much more than this too, as long as you continue to include it with a wide variety of foods from the rainbow – for example, mixed in with the morning porridge, or as a snack on some wholegrain toast. All varieties of nuts have similar health benefits, so include a mixture of peanuts and tree nuts – almonds, walnuts, brazil nuts, cashews, hazelnuts, macadamias, pecans and pistachios – in your child's diet. When they're old enough to eat whole nuts (over five years old; nuts pose a choking hazard if they're any younger), make sure to opt for unsalted varieties that are raw, natural or dry roasted. You'll find many varieties of roasted nuts baked in oil, sugar and salt, making them energy-dense and less nutritious, and these should be avoided.

And lastly, don't buy into the 'activated' scam. Activated nuts are soaked in water for 24 hours and then dried out again so they're still crisp. Despite the clever marketing message, there is no research that activated nuts are better for your child's health or digestion than their natural, raw or dry-roasted counterparts. The only change you will notice is the rise in your grocery bill due to the additional pricing slapped onto the activated products.

When it comes to spreads, if you must include one in your child's diet, butter is better than margarine. But in the ideal world there's no need to buy either of them or to spread them on your child's crackers or other snacks. Extra virgin olive oil and avocado make for great spreads and offer far more nutritional benefits. It might seem crazy at first, but I encourage you to give it a go – you might be surprised that these healthier snacks become something your child loves too.

Healthy, satisfying snacks are an important part of making sure your child's diet is well rounded and balanced. By filling up on these nutritious foods, your child is also less likely to hassle you for sweets and baked goods.

Condiments

Condiments add flavour to a meal, and anything that is tasty is more likely to be consumed by your child. Stock up on some low-salt and low-added-sugar tomato sauce, tomato paste, stock cubes or pre-made stock; most of the time you will use these items in the meal you're cooking rather than as an accompaniment to the dish.

Most other condiments offer little nutritional value and are loaded with empty calories. In an ideal world, they would be left on the supermarket shelves. But, as always, the overall nutrition of your child's meal is more important than the condiment you might be adding to it. If adding aioli or mayonnaise to a sandwich packed with leafy greens and tomato means your child is more likely to eat it, then go for it. What you want to prevent is the situation where your child is saturating every meal with sauce, as any parent who has witnessed a toddler dip a fork in the sauce and avoid the actual food will know! If that happens, they're not getting any flavour from the food itself, which may over time alter their taste preferences and lead to them becoming dependent on condiments for all their meals. Allow them to add a condiment only under your supervision and then put it away and out of sight.

Most condiments are loaded with added fats or added sugars. For example, every dollop of sweet chilli sauce contains 5 teaspoons of added sugar; for teriyaki marinade, it's nearly 3 teaspoons; for tomato sauce, it's 2.2 teaspoons; for tomato chutney, it's 1.2 teaspoons; and for sriracha (hot chilli) sauce it's about 0.8 teaspoons. As for those cleverly marketed fat-free or low-fat salad dressings, you can leave them on the shelves and buy the ordinary full-fat version; the fat-free and low-fat varieties are likely to be higher in added sugar anyway.

Fermented foods

Your child's body contains trillions of bacteria that help them stay healthy, with the majority found in their intestines or gut. Their gut contains both 'good' and 'bad' bacteria, and the balance is largely determined by what they eat. Processed and fast foods will increase the number of bad bacteria in the gut, while high-fibre foods and fermented foods will increase the amount of good bacteria. Fruit, vegetables and wholegrain carbohydrates are important because they are rich sources of fibre and contain prebiotics (which act as a food source for the good bacteria in the gut), and so too are milk-based products and foods that have been fermented (as these contain probiotics that are live microorganisms or good bacteria and exist in the gut to keep it healthy). Prebiotics are the fuel for probiotics and consequently both are needed to increase the population of healthy bacteria in your child's body.

When a food is fermented, it is left to sit until the sugars that the food naturally contains interact with bacteria, yeast and microbes. This process results in an altered chemical structure of the food. Kimchi and sauerkraut are two such examples and are great to include in the family meals. Kimchi is a staple of the Korean diet and there's a lot to be said for that diet when it comes to health – they are one of the leanest populations in the world. However, fermented foods are not for all kids due to their strong flavour, smell and sourness. If your child doesn't yet take to kimchi or sauerkraut, you will find the same good bacteria that you find in fermented foods in milk-based products, such as yoghurt, as well as a fermented sour yoghurt drink called kefir. So, if they don't like the fermented foods, stick to dairy instead.

Tinned and frozen foods

Cooking is time-consuming and can also be very tiresome. This is where both tinned and frozen foods can come into play. Because frozen fruit and vegetables are snap-frozen as soon as they're harvested, they match up nutritionally when compared to their fresh counterparts, and they can save you a lot of time and energy when it comes to preparing the evening meal. Frozen fruit also allows your family to enjoy raspberries and blueberries in the dead of winter, and other veggies that might be out of season, plus they're often cheaper than fresh produce.

Tinned fruit and vegetables also have their benefits. For example, tinned vegetables are pre-cooked, meaning they just need to be heated prior to eating – an excellent time saver in the kitchen. They also have a shelf life of a few years, while frozen vegetables can chill in your freezer for about a year. But tinned vegetables have undergone more processing than frozen versions as the food is heat treated to produce a commercially sterile shelf-stable product with a vacuum seal. They can also contain other additives or ingredients such as salt to increase their shelf life. With respect to tinned fruit, make sure you buy ones in natural juice, not syrup, which is just added sugar.

Irrespective of whether they're fresh, frozen or tinned, there are always nutritional benefits to gain from increasing your child's consumption of fruit and vegetables, so find some they like and expose them to a greater variety over time.

Stock your cupboard with tinned tomatoes, lentils, beans, chick-peas, corn, tuna, salmon, fruit in natural juice and some low-salt vegetable soup. Minced garlic and ginger (no added sugar or salt) are also practical alternatives to avoid relying on fresh produce all the time. But there's no denying fresh garlic and ginger are much more flavoursome. And if you can notice the difference in taste, so will your kids. But this book is all about simplifying your approach to your family's health and making things easier for you, so if this means sticking to the jarred stuff, that is perfectly fine too.

In your freezer, you should stock some frozen vegetables, frozen berries or other fruit, and frozen yoghurt. Frozen pineapple rings, edamame beans and a handful of peas make for great snacks too.

You can also use your freezer as a major meal-prep tool. Produce is cheaper when you buy in bulk, so in our household we often buy the largest packet of chicken breasts or salmon, then divide them up into portions and freeze them in containers until we need them. We're also big fans of doubling a meal and having it for lunch the next day or putting the leftovers in the freezer for another time. Just remember to label the food with the date of cooking so you consume it within a safe time after storage. Fried rice, pasta and risotto all make great freezer meals that children love too. Our toddler is very partial to lentil soup, muffins, homemade pies, spanakopita, dal and bolognaise, all of which you can easily freeze in small portions to have on hand for young children.

Beverages and treats

Milk and water are the only drinks your child needs under the age of two. Breastmilk or formula is all that's required until six months. From six to twelve months, they can also drink cooled, boiled tap water, and this is the time you can start to teach them how to drink from a cup. By the age of 12 months, they can have cow's milk – two cups or 500 millilitres per day is plenty – and they should drink from a plastic cup, not a bottle. Your child does not need fruit juice, soft drink, flavoured or alternative milks or any other beverages.

Even though 100 per cent fruit juice is nutritious and full of naturally occurring sugars, it's far better for your child to enjoy a piece of fruit instead. Eating the whole fruit, rather than only the juice, means they're going to get more fibre as they're consuming the pulp too. So not only is it more nutritious, but it will also fill them up for longer. That's not to say the occasional juice over the age of two is not allowed, it just shouldn't be an everyday occurrence. Once a fortnight is more than enough. Our toddler is a fiend for juice; to avoid a breakfast buffet meltdown on a recent holiday, we watered the juice down to around 20 per cent strength so he could enjoy a treat and we could enjoy a quiet(er) breakfast. It's all about finding the right balance!

Treats include all processed foods. For example, banana bread, chips, ice cream, chocolate and biscuits – pretty much anything you can find in the confectionary or snack aisle in a supermarket – should be considered 'sometimes' foods only. All children (just like adults!) have their favourites, and you need to allow your child to eat their favourite treats occasionally, just not every day. Focus on including treats in your child's diet just once per week – let them choose whatever they want, as long as it's within your budget.

Eating out

Dining out comes down to frequency. From a health point of view, you shouldn't be eating out more than once or twice per week. When you do eat out, don't nitpick at your child's food choices; if they want the burger with chips, allow them to have the burger with chips. A meal you buy at a restaurant or as takeaway will never be as healthy compared to a home-cooked meal, but going out for dinner is not necessarily about health; it's a time to bond as a family, a break from the usual routine and a way to introduce your child to new experiences and foods. It can be a great thing to do, providing you're not doing it all the time. So allow your child to choose their favourite meals when dining out, and, when possible, encourage them to try a range of cuisines. It's also a good idea to try eating out for a mid-week meal when specials can make it more affordable for your family budget, and choose a day in the week when you're more time poor, where having a meal at a restaurant can save you from worrying about food preparation and cooking.

There are also times when you need to make emergency purchases. We've all found ourselves in that situation without food or where we haven't packed enough for our child's needs. Fruit, nuts and dairy products make for great on-the-go snacks that can be quite easy to source when you're out and about, as well as sushi and pre-cut sandwiches.

The benefits of a diet containing animal products

More parents than ever are turning to a vegan diet for a vast range of ethical, cultural and health reasons. This often means they raise their children on the same diet too, which can ring some serious nutritional alarm bells for a growing child.

Veganism is a type of vegetarian diet that means abstaining from all animal products. This means no meat, poultry or fish. It also means no animal by-products, such as eggs and dairy. The focus of a vegan diet is on fruit, vegetables, nuts, seeds and legumes. While this can be a healthy lifestyle for adults, as long as you continue to get enough protein, iron and calcium from other food sources, it can be more challenging for your growing child to meet their nutritional requirements for a variety of vitamins and minerals from a vegan diet.

The first two nutrients you need to consider if your child is on a vegan diet are calcium and vitamin D. Both are needed to develop strong bones and to prevent a disease known as osteoporosis, where bones become more prone to fracture. The richest source of calcium is dairy, which is also a bioavailable source of calcium, meaning this nutrient is highly absorbed in the body. However, for children not consuming dairy products, it's best to opt for calcium-fortified soy products, as we discussed earlier in this chapter, as they are the next closest nutritionally complete alternative. Almonds, dark green leafy vegetables and tofu are also good sources of calcium but their bioavailability is not as high, meaning your child will need to eat much more of these food sources to meet their recommended calcium intake. This can be problematic considering it's hard enough to get kids to eat vegetables in the first place. With respect to vitamin D, which helps absorb calcium from the stomach, it is found in animal by-products, including cheese, eggs and the skin of fish. But the best source of vitamin D is sunlight. So, if your child isn't eating foods like cheese and eggs, make sure they're getting their daily sunlight.

The third nutrient that requires special consideration for children is iron. Iron helps transport oxygen around the body, so if your child complains that they're feeling tired, it's likely their iron levels are low. The best source of iron is meat. Meat is a haem (blood) source of iron, meaning it is highly absorbed in the body. There are lots of non-haem sources of iron, including dark green leafy vegetables, fortified cereals, kidney beans, chickpeas, lentils and almonds. But again, just like with calcium, you need to consume much more of these plant-based sources to meet your recommended dietary intake of iron. And don't think spinach will do it – Popeye's legendary love for the green stuff was in fact incorrectly calculated due to a misplaced decimal point!

The fourth important consideration is vitamin B12, which is required for the formation of red blood cells as well as a healthy brain and nervous system. It is only found in animal products – much higher in the animal product itself, rather than a by-product – and it is imperative for healthy body functioning. It is *not* found in plant sources of food and therefore it is vital to choose B12-fortified foods such as breakfast cereals and soy products – soy milk, tofu and miso. Even with an increased intake of B12-fortified foods, it will be difficult to achieve an adequate intake. This is one to check with your general practitioner, as a supplement is recommended for your child if dietary intake is inadequate. And if you are unsure whether your child should be taking a calcium, iron or vitamin D supplement too, consult with your general practitioner; they can perform a blood test to check and advise on the best course of action.

The fifth nutrient of concern is omega-3 – an essential fatty acid required for a healthy brain. Fish is a rich source of omega-3 fatty acids, and eicosapentaenoic acid (EPA) and docosahexaenoic acid (DHA) are two crucial ones for brain health. Alpha-linolenic acid (ALA) is the plant-based form of omega-3, which is converted to EPA and DHA in the body. However, not all omega-3 fatty acids are created equal, and this conversion process from ALA to EPA and DHA is not that efficient. Again, your child will need more of the plant-based food source to meet their recommended dietary intake of omega-3. EPA and DHA are found in fish, while ALA is found in oil, nuts, seeds and vegetables.

The last consideration is iodine. Iodine is essential for a healthy thyroid, the gland that is the gatekeeper to your child's metabolism and a healthy weight. Iodine is found in the earth's soil, which is then absorbed by the food grown in that soil. But industrial farming practices have resulted in iodine-deficient soils, increasing the risk of iodine deficiency in humans. The richest sources of iodine are fish – found in the skin – and dairy products. Plant-based sources include seaweed, wholegrain bread and beans.

Last, but not least, it is important to note that products labelled 'vegan' are not necessarily healthier than their regular counterparts. Many foods labelled vegan are often highly processed and high in added sugar and fat. It's just ingenious marketing to make it appear as though you are eating a healthier alternative. Anything that is processed is a 'treat' and must be kept in the occasional or sometimes pile.

There are also other types of popular vegetarian diets that can make it much easier for your child to meet their nutritional requirements, rather than adhering to a strict vegan protocol. Pescatarian and flexitarian are two varieties of vegetarian diet that are gaining traction in many households as people choose to move away from eating meat all the time. A pescatarian diet is devoid of meat but allows fish. A flexitarian diet is something we should all be moving towards – it allows for the occasional meat meal, a couple of times per week. It is unlikely your child will be at risk of any nutritional deficiencies if they're eating meat about two times per week.

Lastly, there are three types of vegetarian diets. Lacto-ovo vegetarianism is a diet that includes dairy products and eggs but not meat. Lacto-vegetarian diets include dairy products but not eggs or meat; and ovo-vegetarian diets include eggs but not dairy or meat. It is important that suitable substitutions are made to your child's eating plan if you have them on one of these vegetarian diets.

Dealing with food allergies and food intolerances

Food allergies in children are a major health concern, and they're becoming more common. Food allergies can be very scary. They occur when your child's immune system reacts to an allergen – something in the environment that is normally harmless, such as food proteins. The immune system produces antibodies to the food as if it were a virus or another dangerous foreign invader. This immune system reaction produces allergy symptoms. The most common offenders are egg and peanut, allergies which affect approximately one in ten children under four years of age. Other common causes of food allergy include cow's milk, wheat, soy, fish, shellfish, sesame and other nuts. Understandably, for many parents this can cause a lot of worry and anxiety, particularly if there's a family history of food allergies. Consequently, it's often over-diagnosed by parents, resulting in the unnecessary exclusion of some important food from children's diets, which can have a negative imact on their wellbeing.

Most allergic reactions are mild, but some can be severe. Mild to moderate reactions will present with symptoms such as hives or welts, a tingling feeling in or around the mouth, stomach pain, vomiting and diarrhoea, and facial swelling. A severe reaction, known as anaphylaxis, is a potentially life-threatening situation and requires immediate medical attention. It affects about one in a hundred school-aged children. Symptoms include swelling of the tongue, swelling and tightness in the throat, paleness, floppiness, dizziness, persistent cough, itchy and red skin, and difficulty talking or breathing.

It's easy to confuse a food intolerance with a food allergy, but they're quite different. Even if your child has a reaction to a particular food, it doesn't necessarily mean they have a food allergy. Many children just have intolerances to certain foods. The difference is that a food allergy involves the immune system, while a food intolerance is usually based in the digestive system. Food intolerance will not lead to anaphylaxis as it does not involve the immune system. Intolerance is when your child can tolerate a certain amount of the triggering food, but when you give them too much, they get sick, with symptoms of bloating or diarrhoea in the case of lactose intolerance, for example.

Yes, food allergies are on the rise, but there's plenty you can do to reduce the chances of your child getting one or developing one later in life. The only way to find out if your child is allergic is to give them a range of different foods, particularly the common allergy triggers I mentioned earlier. To avoid any complications, introduce them slowly and monitor for potential reactions. If there is a family history of allergies, this should be done in consultation with your doctor.

Common allergens, such as egg and peanut, should be introduced in the first year of your child's life, around four to six months, or when they are developmentally ready to eat solids. These governing guidelines are the same for all children, even if there's a family history, because studies have shown that introducing known allergens as early as possible helps children develop a tolerance to these foods, as early exposure through the gut can be preventive. Your child will have a lower risk of developing an allergy to foods like egg and peanut the earlier they are provided – specifically an 80 per cent reduction in developing an allergy with early intake.

Start gradually and introduce just a small amount of these foods initially, one at a time. A quarter of a fingernail or a quarter of a teaspoon is a good starting point. For peanut butter, start with just a smear on the inside of their lip. Then monitor your child for 30 minutes. If there is no allergic reaction, you can double the quantity and continue to monitor them for a further 30 minutes. If all goes well, you should continue to include the food in your child's diet in gradually increasing amounts at least weekly.

If your child does have a reaction, it's important not to panic. Mild or moderate allergic reactions (swelling of the lips, eyes or face, or vomiting) can be treated using non-sedating antihistamines such as loratadine. If there are symptoms of anaphylaxis (difficult or noisy breathing, pale skin and floppy limbs, or a swollen tongue) treat with an epinephrine injection (EpiPen) if one is available and call an ambulance immediately. If your child develops a food allergy, it may require ongoing management with a medical professional; your child can grow out of it with time.

CHAPTER 4

MEALTIME, FEELIN' FINE

In the 1950s, over 90 per cent of families in developed countries had their evening meal together sitting around a table. By 2024 this figure has become less than 40 per cent. This is a problem for two reasons. The first one is to do with interaction. Families need a designated time every day when they are interacting with each other, with food as the centre point. It's important because it teaches kids about food, as well as allowing them to enjoy the social benefits of eating and spending time together. The second reason is to do with consumption; by sitting down and eating as a family, we are exposing ourselves to our innate appetite regulation, as the slower mealtime gives our brain time to tell us we are full. Seated family mealtimes at the dinner table, last between 30 and 40 minutes on average, whereas a TV dinner lasts 8 to 12 minutes. The window is shorter for families with very small children – at least that's the case at our place at dinner! – but the point stands, and the significance of this on our digestive system should not be underestimated. Another thing to consider is the difference in food choices that often take place in the two different settings. It's much quicker and easier to grab a microwave meal or takeaway and scoff it down while sitting on the couch, but it will always be far less nutritious and filling than the home-cooked meal you're more likely to serve your family at the dinner table. This is why mealtime is one of the key components of your child's relationship with food. For shift workers, a family breakfast or lunch is also an option, but the key is to do the same thing every day.

Introducing food to a young child is a daunting task. I won't lie; the patience required for a busy parent as they navigate the fussiness and complaints of most children is an exercise in and of itself. But don't force your child to sit at the table until their veggies are finished, no matter how tempting it might be; it is crucial that food is not seen as a punishment or associated with the parent's frustrations and reprimands. It's equally important that food does not become a reward, so don't offer your child a piece of chocolate if they eat their fruit, for example. Data increasingly shows that this is one of the fundamental platforms for your child's relation-ship with food all the way through to adulthood; they'll either associate mealtime as a painful process or a joyful and exciting time, depending on the experiences you give them.

Once you, as the parent, have accepted the importance of positive mealtime experiences, the work begins. Put down the phone, close the laptop, turn off the TV and get stuck in. Sit with your child at mealtimes – to supervise them and to have a healthy snack or a meal at the same time. These day-to-day rituals of eating together will teach them how to eat, as well as how to interact with others, the importance of table manners and how to share food. This way you are modelling good habits, and over time it will lead to your child copying what you do. It will also give you a moment to pause, requiring you to chill out about the mess in the kitchen, food waste and time wasted making gourmet rissoles that nobody ate.

Breakfast as the biggest meal of the day

Setting your child up for success starts with breakfast. As time poor and sleep deprived as we are first thing in the morning, you must pay attention to your child's food intake at their first meal of the day. Preparation, either the night before or as part of a larger weekly meal-prep session, can help ensure you provide your child with sufficient portions, nutrition and variety at breakfast. It doesn't have to be laborious. A nutritious breakfast is actually the easiest meal to put together with smallest amount of time. A tub of yoghurt with some fruit and nuts could do the trick, or wholegrain toast with avocado, a bowl of porridge with 100 per cent nut butter warmed for 60 seconds in the microwave, or some muesli with honey and berries that you prepared the night before.

It's important to engrain this habit of eating breakfast early on in childhood. Why? As we discussed earlier, our bodies use the calories from food more efficiently at the start of the day compared to the end of the day – in fact, 250 per cent more efficiently – due to our circadian rhythm (our natural body clock). Consequently, those who include breakfast every day are better able to manage their body weight throughout adulthood. We have it all wrong in the modern-day Western lifestyle. Breakfast is the most important meal of the day, yet we devote little to no attention to it. We've all been there: we wake up, present our child with a bowl of processed cereal, grab a coffee and then rush off to work, often forgetting to eat anything ourselves. Not only does this leave your child ravenous not long after eating, but it also has a flow-on effect for their day, and you are instilling poor food habits from an early age. Research even shows that the regular inclusion of breakfast is positively associated with academic performance in children. But the benefits of including breakfast extend beyond better performance and behaviour at school. Breakfast consumption is associated with positive outcomes for diet quality, micronutrient intake, weight status and a healthy lifestyle. Focusing on dinner as the largest meal of the day is the wrong way to orientate your child's food intake, as well as your own.

Preparing for the day

The next step in ensuring success at mealtimes is food preparation. A good food-prep routine will help you dodge the dreaded 'convenience eating' hurdle. This is something my patients always complain about – that is, they can never find any good food options on the road when driving their child or children around. The modern-day environment ensures this; there is no shortage of fast food, and it is very challenging to find healthy options when you're on the go. Not to mention the high cost if you do buy food while you're out and about. It's a good idea to take food with you as you leave home every day (for you and your kids); this is the only way to ensure success. If you take your own food and continue to offer it to your child, you will not need to look for convenience food from the drive-through, the park kiosk or the vending machine. For small children, who can quickly become ratty when they're hungry, frequently asking them if they are hungry and providing healthy snacks at regular intervals is the way to go. It's much better to get ahead of the situation and prevent the hunger pangs from creeping in, which only results in tantrums. Older children (5 to 12 years) only need one nutritious snack between meals. Snacking itself is not the problem; it's natural, and only becomes an issue if your child is consuming a bunch of processed foods that aren't filling and that offer little nutritional value. Avoid snacking for the hour before main meals, though, to ensure your child has a better appetite at mealtimes.

Good snacks that don't take much preparation and transport well include: yoghurt; chopped fruit; a piece of bread or wholegrain crackers with avocado, hummus or 100 per cent nut-based spread; a handful of nuts (something like dry-roasted almonds or cashews is ideal); or some chopped-up carrots or cucumber with hummus or guacamole. If you have enough time on the weekend, another winning option is to mass bake snacks and freeze them. Some good options include lentil pies, banana pancakes and homemade cheese-and-tomato scrolls. Some great healthy snack recipes are included in Part 2 of this book, and you can find other recipe suggestions at feedingfussykids.com. Making your own snacks is also significantly cheaper than store-bought options and ensures you can control what goes in them – and your kid.

Placing an emphasis on food intake and preparation at the start of the day is especially important when your child starts school and begins to make their own food choices without your constant supervision. Healthy eating habits begin at home. You, as the parent, have a huge responsibility in setting the right example, providing healthy food options and building a routine that encourages healthy eating. In doing so, you're helping both your child and yourself, as you'll be healthier and filled with energy too – a win for the whole family. Providing your child with a healthy breakfast and packing a healthy lunch are the best ways to make sure they have the energy they need to get through a busy day. Get them involved in packing the lunchbox and ask them what they'd like to eat. If they're engaged in the process, they're also more likely to eat it than throw it out. Leaving them to their own devices at school will only see them stocking up on party pies, chicken nuggets, flavoured milk and custard tarts, all of which are still commonly found in school canteens and frequently mislabelled as 'healthy'.

Meal planning, not diet plans

Food preparation goes hand in hand with meal planning for the week. But this doesn't mean following a calorie-controlled diet or diet plan for your family – you can throw them out. Meal planning just means you need to plan what evening meals you are going to eat for the week and buy the ingredients in advance.

As I mentioned earlier, the best news is that you don't have to cook separate meals for you and your child. Everyone in the household can enjoy the same food, and you can still cook all those family favourites and simple meals that you enjoy cooking. After you read this book, I hope the difference will be that you'll increase the range of foods you're offering your child, as well as upping the nutritious value of easy family favourites like spaghetti bolognaise, pasta bake, tacos, and the classic meat and three veg. Meal planning doesn't need to be complicated, but you do need to focus on variety to ensure your child is regularly exposed to and trialling new foods. This doesn't mean endlessly cooking new recipes; what it does mean is switching it up during the week. An example of a week's worth of dinner plans might look like this:

Monday: Vegetarian enchiladas

Tuesday: Barbecued chicken wraps with salad

Wednesday: Beef hamburger patties with salad (leftover from last night)

Thursday: Slow-cooker chicken and veggies

Friday: Toasted sandwiches

Saturday: Barbecued rissoles with potato chips and greens

Sunday: Oven-baked risotto

This might look daunting, but it's easier to pull together than it seems. The enchiladas, hamburger patties and rissoles can all be made in advance and stuck in the fridge or freezer; if you do take the time to make any of these, make a double batch and freeze half for the future. The salad from Tuesday's wraps can also be eaten with Wednesday's beef hamburger patties (and both can in fact be pre-prepared bags of fresh salad from the supermarket), and toasted sandwiches for Friday is a ten-minute job. Thursday's meal can be cooked with zero input from you after you chuck the chicken and veggies into the slow-cooker, then go about your day.

Your family's meals will be dictated by your schedules, your tastes and how pressed you are for time, but a weekly menu like this is a good way to start meal planning. You should also get your child involved in the meal-planning process when they're old enough, showing them photos of the recipes you will be cooking throughout the week. The leftovers from these meals can also be used for lunch every day, for yourself and/or your child.

As discussed earlier, meal planning and healthy eating is not about restricting your child's food intake, but rather increasing their consumption of wholesome, nutritious foods so, in fact, they end up eating more, not less. Fixating on calorie-controlled meal plans or counting the number of calories your child is eating can have negative long-term consequences on their physical and psychological health. An anxious, calorie-conscious parent will only pass on those negative food associations and habits to their child.

The body is far more complex than it simply being a matter of 'calories in' versus 'calories out', and the body adjusts its metabolic rate based on how much food it is fed. To reiterate what I discussed in the first principle of this whole family approach, it's about *health, not weight* – if you're worried about your child's weight or you've been told to do something about your child's weight, dieting, diet plans and calorie counting are *not* the answer. To be blunt, calorie counting is a complete waste of time and there is nothing to be gained from meticulously recording your child's calorie intake in a smartphone app. You will find not only huge errors in some of the reported calories in foods, but also that, more importantly, all calories are different. One classic example is nuts. As we covered in chapter 3, we don't absorb all the calories in nuts, and they're packed with fibre, ensuring good bowel health for your child. Better still, because they're incredibly filling, a child who just ate some nuts won't nag you for processed snacks. So even though nuts are a source of fat, albeit a good source of fat, their calorie content is not an accurate reflection of what your child's body is absorbing. Vegetables are the same. With their high fibre content, a lot of the calories, particularly in uncooked fruit and vegetables, make their way to the large intestine undigested and they are therefore not absorbed in the body. They're the exact foods you should be providing your child in unlimited amounts, not restricting.

By focusing on the foods that are outlined in the third principle – *the full rainbow* – you will see a natural reduction in the number of calories that your child is consuming, without even focusing on the numbers. More importantly, you will be providing the nutrition and satisfying food your child's body needs to ensure proper growth and development.

A good template to follow for your child's meals is to include a lean protein source, a wholegrain carbohydrate, a source of good fat and plenty of salad or vegetables. Examples of this include beef and vegetable pie, chicken and salad wraps, meat pasta with vegetables, and tofu stir-fry. If you follow this guideline, you will never put a foot wrong. The tricky part is getting your child to eat this nutritious food. But, over time, as you implement the principles of this plan and embrace this whole family approach, you will see an improvement in your child's eating habits and less resistance to the healthy foods you serve.

Mealtime rules

As a parent, it's important to create boundaries and structure around mealtimes, so you minimise having to negotiate and argue with your child. To address this, here are some simple rules for you and your child that should form the basis of every mealtime.

1. Eat as a family

Wherever possible, meals should be eaten around the dining table. This is especially important when it comes to the evening meal. Dinner is the most important meal from a social and cultural perspective – it's a time to reflect on your day and engage with others at the table. This is especially relevant if you have an infant or toddler as they will absorb and adopt your behaviour from a very early age. There are no individual meals; instead, everyone sits together and eats the same thing, including the six-month-old (who is, in fact, developmentally ready to do so).

Setting the table is the first step. If they're old enough, it's a simple task and responsibility that your child can complete each day. From three years old, children are capable of taking the cutlery (but be mindful of the knives) or condiments over to the table and returning them to the kitchen at the end of the meal. There should also be no distractions at the table – no TV (not even running in the background), laptops, phones or other electronic devices. Mealtime is family time.

In saying this, dinner is a stressful event for many households. Despite the toddler throwing most of their food on the floor, the children arguing at the table or the complaints that they don't like the food, the one thing you need to do is sit together as a family. Not only does it help everyone be mindful of what they are eating but it also sets a good example by making mealtime a daily ritual.

And remember that children model your behaviour, so you need to be consistent in your approach. In a two-parent family, it's important to support one another and not undermine the other's activities, otherwise all the good work of one will be undone by the other.

You will get better outcomes if your child is hungry right before mealtimes, so make sure they aren't filling up on snack food for one to two hours before. You're also likely to get better outcomes at dinnertime if your child eats their evening meal early – before 6 p.m. – because they are more likely to eat well when they're not tired. This often means only one parent will be present due to work–life demands, but if you can squeeze in a couple of nights per week where you are all together, the results with respect to your child's food acceptance will be even better.

2. Encourage them to try new foods

It's not uncommon for a child to be particularly set on only eating one type of food and to avoid trying new foods. If you find yourself in this position, make sure not to offer this favourite food all the time – at first, only offer it every second day and in a variety of different ways. You can even nominate a day of the week when they can have their favourite food. If you want your child to like healthy foods, they need repeated, positive experiences with such foods from an early age, and ample opportunity to see others eat them too. Children are more likely to try a new food if an adult eats it first. When you present your child with a new food, simply ask them to try it. This sets a clear boundary for your child's behaviour. It's important not to bribe, beg or reward to get them to try something new, and you must avoid giving in to that temptation. Instead, simply ask and encourage them to try the new food. You can let them decide whether they like it or not, and they don't have to finish it – just try it.

If you run out of one food that you know your child loves, try offering a similar alternative. For example, if they love melon and you only have peaches, offer the peaches to your child. When they ask what it is, just answer 'fruit' rather than specifying the actual fruit. You don't want to give them the opportunity to tell you they don't like it before they've even tasted it. But don't try to sell it as something it's not.

Talk about healthy food in a positive manner – 'these carrots are yummy' – rather than forcing it on your child. Family mealtimes offer you a chance to eat it in front of them, and if they decide to leave it, this is fine. Same goes if they refuse to eat their dinner, but demand dessert. Again, don't force them to eat their dinner and promise them dessert if they do. Research has proven that using unhealthy foods as a reward will only increase your child's preference for them, which makes it even harder to wean them off the junk. Tell them they need to eat dinner before dessert and explain why – a gentle way to remind your child that certain foods are better for our health than others, without bribing them or saying a particular food is 'bad'. Another way of describing the difference between the two is that our body relies on everyday foods – like the meal on the table – for healthy growth and development, but it doesn't need 'sometimes' foods – dessert – in the same way. As we covered in the second principle – *reach for nature first* – it's also a good idea to serve nature's treats like chopped fruit as dessert and to limit the 'sometimes' foods to just once per week.

Most often your child's stubbornness around only eating one favourite food is to do with their developmental need for control; they are simply testing your limits to see if they can get what they want. Unfortunately, you may need to offer a new food multiple times before they try it. In fact, research shows that you need to offer a food about seven times before you get success. That's a lot of carrots on the floor! But don't lose hope – keep trying and encouraging them to give it a go.

3. Add variety to your family favourites

You can make the same meals often but try to introduce different flavours every time. While variety in our weekly meals is important, it's also important not to overdo it. As you continue offering your child small quantities of new foods, you're probably going to get less resistance from them if you serve up slightly different variations of the same thing. For example, if your child is familiar with bolognaise, you might try a beef version on one occasion and a lentil bolognaise the next.

There still needs to be a degree of familiarity with the food on the table to encourage your child to try new foods, but there are many ways you can put a slightly different spin on a family classic. Instead of beef meatballs, try making them with chicken mince; instead of plain chicken breasts, try adding different herbs or lemon before baking. You can also try mixing up the vegetables you add to different dishes or add different fruits to sweet dishes (for example, pancakes). If your child finds raw carrots too confronting, try our trick – stick them in the oven and serve 'orange chippies'. Another good way to get vegetables into a reluctant toddler (or adult!) is to grate them and add them to meatballs, pasta sauces or pies.

4. Bring the fun back into food

As with the 'orange chippies', you'll spark your child's interest when you give healthy recipes fun names, and if you let your child eat fruit and vegetables in the way they prefer. For example, some children prefer tinned fruit (remember to only buy the kind in natural juice) or raw chopped vegetables, while others prefer frozen fruit and cooked veggies. One of our children is a fiend for 'cold berries' but isn't partial to the same fruit fresh. Some children also like their fruit cut in small bite-sized pieces and many like it to be cut up in shapes or objects. The same can be said for mealtimes; your child is more likely to be interested in food that has different shapes and colours – food that is visually appealing, as you will find with many recipes in this book and at feedingfussykids.com.

Child-friendly plates and utensils can also make a difference. Go shopping with your child and allow them to choose their favourites. It may also be beneficial to eat in different areas of the home, such as outdoors – this will break the normal routine and can be the required spark needed to get your child to eat and enjoy the food experience. The occasional dinner picnic is good for everyone.

5. Educate your child on the science of food

Getting your child or children to grow their own herbs and vegetables is educational and a great way of getting them interested in the food they eat. They'll have lots of fun partaking in the gardening process too. The same can be said for food shopping; children will get a lot of joy out of seeing the wide range of fresh fruit and vegetables at the fruit shop, the different types of fish at the fishmonger's and the wide variety of meat at the butcher's. And just like cooking, these activities shouldn't wait until they reach school age. Instead, you should get your child involved as early as possible. Many children also benefit from being read books about food or listening to music about food.

When it comes to gardening, it doesn't need to be difficult; depending on the amount of space you have available, a small, raised garden bed on your verandah or a tomato plant from the supermarket on the windowsill is perfectly fine. Asking your child to look after the plant is a simple task that will give them an understanding and appreciation of how food is grown and teach them responsibility through caring for the plant. It will also develop their love of nature – time outside is always better than time spent in front of the television – and build their self-confidence through enjoying the food they have grown. Plus, there is a lot to be learnt about the science of growing your own food. Simple, fun facts about different foods your child grows is another aspect of teaching them the basics of nutrition and why some foods are better for them than others.

Children of different ages will have different expectations and experiences when it comes to this sort of education. Suitable tasks for toddlers include watering plants, pulling out weeds, harvesting produce and planting new seedlings, whereas older children can help you dig, plant and prune. Younger children also get a lot of joy out of making the garden a fun space, such as making a scarecrow, having a water feature or building a worm farm if you have the space.

The science of food is not just limited to the growing of it. It's important to teach your child the basics of what each food offers as well (as you would when grocery shopping too). Younger children and toddlers benefit more from sensory education – try giving them a freshly harvested vegetable to hold and ask them if it is soft or crunchy, dry or wet. Older children benefit from more direct nutritional education, which can be presented as fun food facts at mealtimes. Some examples include:

- Fish is packed with a special type of fat called omega-3 to make us smarter.
- Potatoes are packed with vitamins and minerals that keep us healthy.
- Chicken is high in protein which helps build strength (with accompanying Popeye arm gestures, of course!).

- Cheese is made from milk, which is high in calcium to form strong bones.
- Beans are packed with fibre to keep our tummy healthy.
- Fruits and vegetables are loaded with vitamins and minerals to stop us from getting sick.

Remember to use age-appropriate language and teach them why food matters.

6. Involve them in cooking

Cooking is a time to involve the children before you all sit down to a meal together. Believe it or not, kids love to cook. In fact, they love to do anything you're doing. And the easiest way to get them involved in the kitchen is by giving them simple tasks to make them feel part of the cooking process. For example, mixing ingredients together, mashing or tipping ingredients into a bowl, or pulling basil leaves off the stem are things that even a toddler can do. And because they've contributed to the meal, they're more likely to try it when you sit down to eat as they'll be proud of what they've made. You don't need to wait until your child starts high school to be doing this. You can have them participate in cooking at home from as early as two years of age. You can also buy toddler-specific cutting knives if you're game.

How much food should you serve your child at mealtimes?

You should let your child dictate how much they wish to eat. A one-year-old will still be quite dependent on you feeding them, but by age two they can feed themselves with their hands, and by age three they can use utensils. You should always watch your child while they're eating to avoid choking accidents, especially when they're under the age of five. For the same reason, they shouldn't eat in the car.

When it comes to the quantity of food, take note of what your child eats in a week, rather than at one meal or in one day. Half of the success lies in parental perception. The portions you, or your older children eat, are no point of comparison to the small amounts of food a toddler needs to eat, so don't be concerned when they don't finish everything on their plate. As I mentioned in chapter 2, many millennial parents will remember being forced to finish their dinner – don't do this to your own children. It's best to serve up less food than you think they need, with a focus on variety. Allow your child to experiment and present them with the same food the whole family is eating. If your child asks for more at one meal, don't necessarily expect the same for the next meal – this is nothing to worry about. They'll compensate across the course of the day and a week. If food is available constantly, they will eat enough to fulfil their needs, but when food is not available or to their taste, they will compensate by eating more when it is. Also, how they eat in one day doesn't reflect how they will eat the next. Don't be surprised if the risotto they loved on Sunday is public enemy number one by Monday, or if something they eat with friends or at school is rejected at home.

It just takes one good meal a day to help keep your young child healthy and nourished, and for them to experience the benefits of family mealtime, so don't think you'll get success at every sitting. It's worth considering that your child may eat a wide variety and large amount of food at kinder or day care, and then they refuse to eat at home that evening. At least they're eating healthy food somewhere! Your child will know when they are full. There is no need to force them to finish the plate or bowl of food. They self-regulate their food intake according to a complex process involving both the gut and brain. Remember, it's the child who determines how much breastmilk or formula they consume at each feed, not the parent. Young infants and children only eat what they need. A small child will tell you when they are full, verbally or through other signals: they will turn their head away from the fork or spoon; they will close their lips when food is presented to their mouth; they will push the bowl or plate away with their hand; or they will shake their head or say they don't want any more. The opposite is also true: when they are hungry, they will get excited; they'll make noises when they see food; they will place their hands near their mouth; they will lean towards you when you have food; or they will open their mouth when you feed them. And when they're old enough (from two years of age), they will tell you when they're hungry. Simple signs of communication.

What do I do with leftovers?

It's very common for your child to leave leftovers; they will a lot of the time. Don't make them eat everything on their plate or provide rewards for eating their food. Instead, ask them if they're still hungry, and if they're content, cover and put the leftovers in the fridge for later, or throw them out. Of course, it is better to prevent food wastage as much as possible, and we freeze all our scraps for the neighbouring chooks. This is where a worm farm can also come in handy to complement your veggie garden.

I know it's very tempting to eat your child's leftovers or to pinch a mouthful of food while they eat; you might want to prevent wasting food, but this form of mindless eating can be due to many factors, such as stress, boredom, hunger, lack of sleep and mindlessness. It's called the 'if it's there, you'll eat it' phenomenon and it can be a challenging habit to break, particularly towards the end of the day. But for you as a parent, the biggest rule you need to follow for your own health is to not eat your child's leftovers, as it can result in unnecessary weight gain. Ideally, you should eat at the same time as your child, but do it by serving up your own plate or bowl of food.

Tips for when life gets in the way

There is no questioning the demands of modern-day life on parents. You may be juggling work with kids, or you may be very busy as a stay-at-home parent, which often means the end of the day can be the most challenging. The last thing you'll feel like doing is cooking, and the thought of takeaway or fast food is very appealing.

But rather than defaulting to the easy option of ordering in, it's a hundred times better to grab a barbecue chicken and a bag of salad from the supermarket, or to put together something simple, such as an omelette on wholegrain bread, or a toasted sandwich or flatbread. You might even find some leftovers in the freezer that can save the day, or you can stock your freezer with things like frozen fish fillets, chicken schnitzel and bags of vegetables like peas. The occasional fish finger is also fine to keep on hand, but these should be saved for a treat and not a daily occurrence, as we covered in chapter 3. Fish fingers are processed fish products that have been battered and breaded. Frozen fish fillets, on the other hand, are a cheaper alternative to fresh fish; they are fresh fish that has been frozen at time of capture, and therefore their nutrition is retained.

On the days when you are cooking, aim to cook more food or a double batch so that you and your family have leftovers for the following day and have stocked the freezer for emergencies. You can also chop extra veggies and store them in your crisper, ready to use for the next meal or snack. As we don't have time to prepare all family meals from scratch every day, utilising leftovers for lunch is a perfect way to ease some of the burden around meal planning and will reduce the frequency of eating out or having to give your child money to buy food from the school canteen. The last thing we have time for in the morning is preparing meals for the day. It's hard enough getting the kids ready. Leftovers alleviate this stress and pain and will help you keep the whole family on track for a healthier diet and lifestyle.

CHAPTER 5

PLAY EVERY DAY

The ability to walk on two legs is one of the earliest defining features of human evolution, one that came about around six million years ago. We need movement to survive. But while nomadic and hunter-gatherer tribes continue this tradition, humans living in modern urbanised society have drastically removed it from daily life. Mostly we use motorised transport for getting about – cars, trains or buses. To walk a kilometre for milk is not something we're likely to do. Yet we hear of great distance runners from Kenya, Ethiopia and Tanzania, who explain their incredible feats of fitness as a result of having had to run 20 kilometres to school and back every day. Today's children, at least those living in modern Western civilisations, take on average less than 6000 steps per day. On short legs, this is less than 4 kilometres per day. Many of us parents sit in an office for large chunks of the day, while our kids sit for hours at school. And when the family returns home, they'll probably end up sitting in front of the TV for most of the evening.

This acceptance of non-movement has become part of our modern programming. Consequently, physical inactivity is now a leading cause of early death. And this sedentary lifestyle starts on day one in the home, in the habits that are instilled in children by their parents. Children do not see their parents moving; consequently, they do not move. We are programming them to think that exercise and physical activity is optional or something we need to do in a gym or in a game of sport, when in reality humans evolved to walk long distances and hunt for food as part of a nomadic lifestyle – not a lifestyle in which we place our children in front of screens and teach them to turn on gadgets for everything from entertainment to education.

Our sedentary lives are killing us early, and they're setting children up for a lifelong struggle with not only their weight but also, more importantly, their health. But by embracing this principle of the whole family approach – *play every day* – you can help your child be more active, and activity will become a central part of their life and yours.

What does the research show?

When it comes to how much exercise our children are doing, it doesn't bode well. Only one in three children aged two to seventeen years of age are meeting the physical activity guidelines for their age group. The guidelines vary but, simply put, those aged less than one year should do plenty of floor play at short, frequent intervals. From one to five years of age they should be physically active for at least three hours per day, while children aged five to eighteen years should do at least one hour of moderate to vigorous physical activity each day, plus several hours of light physical activity or incidental exercise each day. For those aged five to eighteen years of age, at least three days a week should include activities that strengthen muscles and bones, such as jumping, running and climbing.

By way of example, the following sections are a summary of what your child's activities might look like across the course of the day, broken up by age group. On the days they attend day care or preschool, it's often very easy to achieve. But on the other days, a more conscious effort is needed from you as the parent to make sure they are getting enough movement in their life.

Infants (birth to 1 year)

Promoting child movement and tummy time is an important part of development. You should start tummy time for your child soon after birth, beginning with one- to two-minute sessions, up to four times per day. They don't like it, but don't give up – it's important to keep trying! Placing your child on their stomach encourages them to flex and strengthen their head and neck muscles, important for their overall physical development, and it helps prevent any flat spots on their head. By four to six months, active play is as important for your child as food and sleep. Getting them to reach for and grasp objects will engage them more in the activity. Supervised tummy time should increase to at least ten minutes, three times a day at six months (totalling thirty minutes), and they'll be increasingly active as they begin to crawl and walk – important milestones for their motor development, muscle strength and coordination.

Toddlers (1 to 2 years)

Physical activity for toddlers should be fun. The more active they are, the better. They need at least three hours of exercise of varying intensity spread across the course of the day. This can be achieved by playing ball games with your child or racing each other at the park, going for short bushwalks, playing at the playground and dancing to music, to name a few examples. All of these activities get you involved too, boosting your own movement.

Preschoolers (3 to 5 years)

Preschoolers also need at least three hours of physical activity each day, including one hour of energetic play, which includes things like free play at the pool, riding a bike, playing ball games, climbing at the playground and running around with friends (or you!) in the backyard or at the park. Children at this age are learning to hop, skip and jump, and they're eager to show off how they can kick or throw a ball, do a cartwheel, or balance on one foot. Join in and encourage them to do so.

Getting involved in organised sport is not required for pre-schoolers. They're still learning the basics of catching, kicking, throwing and taking turns. Simple rules may be hard for them to understand. If you do get them involved, make sure it's age appropriate and one that focuses on fun and understanding the fundamentals of the sport, rather than anything competitive or highly structured. Otherwise, it can wait until they reach school.

School-aged children and teenagers

During primary school years it's important to focus on fun game-based formats, not drills. Get them to trial a wide range of sports and focus on a couple that they really like. As they grow up, the emphasis in sport shifts to a more adult, winning-focused style. Some children and teenagers certainly enjoy this competition, but others will prefer other styles of activity.

If you notice your child or teenager isn't enjoying sport anymore, encourage different ways to be active. This might involve changing sports, changing teams or coaches, or partaking in recreational exercise rather than structured sport. Anything to keep them engaged in regular exercise is a win as they will still get the physical and mental health benefits without a focus on competition and pressure to win.

Playing sport and partaking in physical activity during these years will continue to provide lifelong benefits to your child's physical, mental and social wellbeing. If they grow up with exercise engrained in their day-to-day life they're also more likely to remain active as adults and to have improved resilience and social connectedness.

Daily movement

Unfortunately, most of us are sedentary. Therefore, the focus when it comes to exercise needs to be on making gradual but realistic and sustainable changes that become a way of life. As with strict diets, adopting an all-or-nothing approach to movement will not stick long term and can result in injury. Your child learns from you, so incorporating regular daily movement in your family's routine will encourage them to be active throughout childhood and adulthood, making those healthy habits stick. Incidental exercise is just as important as structured physical activity, so as a first point of action, think of ways you can get the whole family moving. Some habits you can implement include:

- walking or riding your bikes to school or the shops instead of driving
- using the stairs instead of a lift
- parking at the back of the supermarket car park to incorporate walking to and from your car
- getting off the bus one stop earlier than your usual stop
- catching public transport instead of driving

- using social catch-ups as an opportunity for exercise by meeting friends at the park or the pool, or going for a walk together
- tackling the gardening or housework as a family.

Structured physical activity

Once you have made adjustments to include incidental or opportune movement in your family's lifestyle, it's important to then incorporate regular structured physical activity every day. The hardest thing for people who have been non-movers for most of their lives can be overcomplicating or overthinking the type of physical activity they should be doing, when a simple walk, kicking a ball, going for a bike ride or swimming will suffice. It's not about ribbons, awards, medals and accolades; it's about putting in place a pattern whereby your child actually seeks out movement and exercise because it has become a habit. The neural pathways formed in their brain from this regular, repeated behaviour will naturally steer them towards that way of life – one where exercise and physical activity is intertwined in their day-to-day life.

All physical activities are great. The most important thing is to participate in the ones your child enjoys. It's also valuable to trial new things and to explore different environments, so be sure to offer a variety of different activities to your child. But this doesn't mean going to places you can't afford or taking your child to environments that are not appropriate. You don't have to sign them up to soccer, netball and swimming lessons, or any of the many activities that come with sign-up fees and extra costs like uniforms and travel expenses. Children love free play. They don't need structured activities like organised sport until they commence school – and even then, they may still prefer recreational activity! The local playground is a classic for a reason.

How to get kids moving

The goal is to get your child moving, and the best encouragement comes from doing. If you're seen to be regularly moving, they're more likely to move too. From a young age, family time together should be spent on fun fitness activities, not strict exercise regimes such as going to the gym. Fun and enjoyment is paramount to setting up a positive association with movement for your child. Take them to the park to play on the equipment; kick or throw different balls at the oval; head to the beach and look for crabs, build a sandcastle or swim; go for a bushwalk; run around with them or make an obstacle course in your yard if you have the room; play some music and have a dance party at home; or play hopscotch on your driveway. Anything to encourage activity and get them moving. If you're stuck inside, set up a safe area with an obstacle course made out of boxes and chairs for your child to go over, under and around, play volleyball with a balloon, or set up a treasure hunt throughout your home with a list of items to find.

Children don't need fancy devices or wearables to measure their activity levels. Despite the rise in popularity in wearable technology, tracking steps and movement could have negative consequences in children and can trigger obsessive behaviour, particularly when many tracking devices encourage users to share their results with friends. Children also engage in activity for different reasons, both in the nature of the activity and their motivators for participating in it. So, instead of focusing on how much they're doing, provide them access to parks, playground equipment and outdoor spaces where they can run and play. This is the best way of increasing their movement!

Exercise during pregnancy

Physical activity is not just important for your child's health, it's vital for you too, but it becomes harder to find time if it's your second or third pregnancy and you already have a child. Nevertheless, pregnancy represents one of the greatest physical challenges you will ever experience and to support these changes to your body, staying physically active is key. And despite what you may think, pregnancy is a time to start moving even if you don't usually exercise.

There are numerous health benefits to gain from exercising during pregnancy. Regular exercise will help you carry the extra weight from your growing child, reduce complications associated with pregnancy, prepare you for the physical challenge of labour and birth, improve your mood and vitality, improve your sleep quality, and help you bounce back quicker to your pre-pregnancy weight following the delivery of your child. But these benefits aren't just limited to you; they extend to your child as well. The prenatal environment – the environment inside the uterus, where the unborn child is developing – plays an unexpected role with respect to exercise too. There's growing evidence that physical activity during pregnancy can influence how well and willingly your child moves on their own. Children born to mothers who exercise during pregnancy develop stronger, more athletic hearts and have accelerated motor development.

You should be aiming for at least 30 minutes of moderate-to vigorous-intensity exercise on most days of the week. But if you haven't been exercising regularly, sudden increases in structured physical activity are *not* advised, and you should get health screened at your general practitioner or primary-care provider if you haven't done any exercise in six months or more. If that's your situation, rather than jumping straight into the recommended 30 minutes of physical activity per day, start gradually with low- to moderate-intensity exercise, gradually increasing the level – for example, try walking for 10 minutes per day and build up to 30 minutes per day over the course of a month. Research has shown that breaking your physical activity up into shorter bouts is just as beneficial for heart health as physical activity undertaken in one long session. Two 15-minute walks are just as good as one 30-minute walk each day. This is because you're more likely and able to work out harder if the duration is shorter.

Sudden increases in the amount of exercise you do will only see you injured, and you may even be putting yourself at risk of heart attack. You're also likely to end up with a very painful muscular side effect called delayed-onset muscle soreness (DOMS). DOMS is nothing to worry about if you do end up with it, but it's very painful and happens when the muscle fibres break down, consequently resulting in a lot of pain even with small movements. You will end up with DOMS if you haven't exercised in a while or if you try a new type of exercise.

As you progress and become able to complete 30 minutes of structured physical activity, you should mix up your routine by including some muscle-strengthening exercises, starting at one day per week and building up to two days per week. Muscle-strengthening exercises can also be as easy as doing something in the comfort of your own home, and you don't need weights. You can use objects in your house, such as water-filled milk bottles, or food tins, and it's also enough to do exercises using your body weight only (such as squats and push-ups).

If you're already a regular exerciser, remember you're growing a person inside you, so it's not a time to reach new fitness heights. Focus on maintaining your current activity level, particularly during the latter stages of pregnancy or second and third trimesters when you start to feel more uncomfortable. Avoid the introduction of new activities and focus on exercising at an intensity you can manage.

What exercises are best during pregnancy?

The best type of exercise is one that gets your heart pumping and makes you sweat, without causing physical distress – walking, cycling or swimming are great if you're first starting out. Running, aqua aerobics, yoga, Pilates, and specific pregnancy exercise classes that your gym may offer are also great aerobic workouts. YouTube also has an endless supply of pregnancy workout videos. If your gym doesn't offer pregnancy-specific classes, be sure to tell the instructor of any class you attend that you are pregnant so they can modify according to your needs.

Exercise needn't follow strict routines; anything that gets you moving is fine. Many people associate exercise with lifting weights, personal training or gym classes. This is perfectly fine if you love going to the gym or being told what to do when it comes to exercise, but don't think that the expense of a gym membership will coax you into attending. The reality is most people stop going two weeks after signing up. Many people don't like the gym environment as it may trigger their lack of self-worth as they begin to compare themselves to other people exercising alongside them, and thinking they're not as slim, fit, strong or toned, they simply give up. Some people also find it too much of a hassle to go somewhere specific to do an activity they aren't especially keen on. The whole notion of getting in your car and driving somewhere to work out is absolute madness. If anything, you should be walking there! This is not to say you should rule out a gym completely, because for many, a gym is everything. Many fitness or recreation centres also offer much more than a gym. Some have pools and childcare facilities too, which can make it easier for you to exercise if you already have a child. But before you sign up, try out a range of different gyms to ensure it is the one for you. Many have free trials allowing you to do so. It doesn't matter if you're looking for a pool to swim laps, gym classes or specific classes devoted to your needs (pregnancy), an area to work out solo if you prefer solitude, a dance class if you danced growing up, and so on; all that matters is that it's the right environment for you.

You should avoid all contact sports, scuba diving and any activities at high altitudes (for example, skiing) during pregnancy. It's also not advised to partake in activities with an increased risk of falling, such as trampolining, gymnastics and horse riding.

You can still lift weights, but you should focus on less resistance with higher repetitions, rather than heavy weights and low repetitions. Beyond 16 weeks it is best to perform exercises while standing, sitting or lying on your side. Exercising on your back can make you feel light-headed.

What intensity should you aim for?

With respect to exercise intensity, the sweat factor is one of the best guides, even for people who don't typically sweat. Increasing your walking speed is a straightforward way to increase the intensity. Unfortunately, not all exercise can involve walking while sipping on a latte and talking to your friend (these are bonus steps you can get instead of sitting in the cafe with the banana bread). When I refer to moderate intensity exercise, this is where you are walking at a pace that makes you huff and puff and that makes you sweat. You can still maintain a conversation, but you will be huffing and puffing as you go.

Put simply, if you are sweating, you are doing it right. But remember that pregnancy is not a time to reach new fitness heights, so exercise within your comfort zone. You can still include high-intensity training, but you will find as your body changes during pregnancy, so does your ability to exercise at higher intensities. This is particularly relevant beyond the 16-week mark of your pregnancy, which is the time to modify your training to focus on continuous, lower intensity exercise. There is certainly benefit in mixing up the type of exercise and intensity through-out pregnancy, but it's more important that you're moving regu-larly, and long-term habits come from partaking in activities you like. As discussed earlier, building activity into your daily life is just as important; gardening, housework, walking between meetings and using the stairs instead of the lift, are all great ways of increasing your incidental activity.

Continuous versus high-intensity interval training

High-intensity interval training, popularly known as HIIT, can also be considered earlier in your pregnancy. For those who are not familiar with the concept of HIIT training, it involves incor-porating bouts of very high intensity (i.e. high heart rate) exercise for short periods of time, followed by periods of low-intensity movement to recover, before repeating another high-intensity burst, and so on, until you complete the prescribed session. For example, you would pedal as hard as you can on a stationary bike (a recumbent bike is perfectly fine) for 10 seconds (the 'on' period), before pedalling slowly for 30 seconds so you can get your breath back (the 'off' period). You keep repeating this 'on' and 'off' period, exercising the whole time, until 15 or 20 minutes is up. Another example is walking: you could walk fast for one minute and then walk at a slower pace for two minutes to catch your breath back, repeating the pattern for a set amount of time (again, it might be 10 or 20 minutes).

HIIT sessions are a wonderful addition to your repertoire of physical activities that you can add to your weekly plan, espe-cially on days when you are time poor. And it doesn't matter what size you are; anyone can do them. But pregnancy is not a time to reach new fitness heights – it's just important that you move every day.

The pelvic floor

The pelvic floor is a group of muscles that support the organs (bladder, uterus and bowel) in your pelvis. It runs from the front of your pubic bone to your sitting bone at the back. If it is weak, gaps start to appear and parts of your bladder or bowel might start descending through them resulting in a leaky bladder or incontinence. The extra weight and force during pregnancy can weaken your pelvic floor.

Specific pelvic-floor stability exercises should be included every day during your pregnancy, because a weak pelvic floor can result in all sorts of barriers to other exercise. It can be hard to identify the right muscles, and the easiest way to test this is when sitting on the toilet for a wee. While midstream, stop the flow and hold for a few seconds – these are the muscles you are targeting. An easy and simple exercise to do every day is the pelvic squeeze. There are two variations of the same exercise that you should do three times a day. While standing, squeeze and lift the muscles as if you're trying to stop a wee. Hold the squeeze for up to five seconds and then relax for five seconds. Repeat 10 times (it will take you less than two minutes to complete). Build up to 10-second holds as your pelvic floor strength increases. Following this, do three sets of 10 quick squeezes, without the 5-second hold (each set will take approximately 10 seconds to complete, so three sets with a 10-second break in between will take you only a minute to complete). The great thing about this exercise is you can do it anywhere – for example, while waiting in the queue to the bus, waiting for your morning coffee, waiting at home for the kettle to boil, or talking to your colleague at work; no one will even know you're doing it.

Preventing injury

If you haven't exercised for a while but want to start doing so for your own health and the health of your unborn child, it's important to start off gradually while keeping the long-term goal at the front of mind. The extra body weight you are carrying during pregnancy will impose undue stress on your joints, which is exacerbated when taking part in certain types of exercise, including walking. You must gradually increase the amount of exercise you do, just like an athlete would gradually increase the amount of training they do. Drastic changes in activity or intensity are not advised.

It is also important to consider non-body-weight-bearing exercise or workouts while seated to alleviate the stress on your joints. Joint pain is a common complaint for a large percentage of the population during pregnancy. In this instance, most incidental exercise will not be practical, and you will only be able to achieve the recommended amount of physical activity through the incorporation of non-body-weight-bearing exercise, such as swimming, cycling and rowing. Recumbent bikes that you can use in the comfort of your own home are particularly good as the seats are comfortable, allowing you to exercise for long periods of time without the common complaint of a sore saddle after riding. Swimming is another great exercise that takes the stress off your joints, as is completing a seated gym routine at home with tins of food as the resistance. It doesn't matter what you do on the bike, in the pool, or in your home gym environment, all that matters is that you move.

Even if body-weight-bearing exercise is fine for you, incorporating a day of non-body-weight-bearing exercise in between each day is advised. For example, walk on Monday (body-weight bearing), ride your bike on Tuesday (non-body-weight bearing), walk again Wednesday (body-weight bearing), go for a swim on Thursday (non-body-weight bearing), do a gym activity on Friday (body-weight bearing), use a rowing machine on Saturday (non-body-weight bearing), and so on. This will give your muscles and joints time to recover between exercise sessions. It will also prevent injury and disappointment from not being able to exercise.

You shouldn't be scared to exercise during pregnancy, but you need to apply some precautions. You should stop exercising whenever you experience any pain, dizziness, light-headedness, weakness, blurred vision, excessive fatigue, shortness of breath before exertion, or vaginal bleeding.

Increase in appetite with exercise

Many people report an increase in hunger following exercise. Despite what the research shows (that this is not usually the case), you need to listen to your body and give it the nutrition it requires. You should never deprive yourself, or the child you are growing, of food. If you feel hungry, you should eat, but always remember to *reach for nature first*. Think of an increase in hunger as your body telling you it is starting to work more efficiently and that it is responding to the new stresses (physical activity) you have introduced. Embrace it, don't fear it!

Exercising with the children around

Some of you will already have a child. Having children presents a wonderful and opportune time to move. There is absolutely no reason why you can't be moving when they are, even if you're pregnant. If they want to play on the playground equipment, play with them. If they want to kick a ball, kick it with them. If they're playing sport, walk around the oval while watching them. Your focus should simply be getting involved with your child or children.

And if that's not appropriate because they're playing with their friends, you can still be exercising nearby, keeping them in sight.

Some other great ways to increase your exercise while pregnant is to walk your child to school, go for family walks after dinner, or ride your bikes instead of driving to the shops. If you find you're playing taxi driver all day, it might not always be practical to walk around the oval or exercise while your child is playing sport. Of course, this is the ideal situation, but if you're dropping Charlotte at one event, Sally at the next and then Eddie 15 kilometres in the other direction, it's not practical to be active when they are. You'll find yourself sitting in the car the whole time. You might be able to team up with another parent or your partner and share the pick-ups and drop-offs, or you might find that you can do a little movement at each drop-off. All those five-minute bursts of activity will add up. Otherwise, try getting up a little earlier in the morning and get some movement in before you leave, or schedule some alone time in the afternoon and take the children out to play later in the day. There is always a way to incorporate exercise into your day, and the children will love it because there is nothing more they want to do than play. As I mentioned earlier, some gyms also offer childcare facilities.

When is it safe to return to exercise after pregnancy?

Exercise will help you recover after childbirth, improve your mood, help prevent postnatal depression and strengthen your muscles. There's plenty you can do to get your body moving but how soon until you can start moving will depend on your individual circumstances. It will also depend on how active you were before you had the baby and what sort of delivery you had (vaginal or caesarean).

After a vaginal birth, you can start gentle walking when you feel up to it. Build up gradually until you can walk for 30 minutes.

Within a day or two of birth, you should also recommence the pelvic squeeze activity I described earlier, provided there is no increase in your pain. As your body goes through big changes with pregnancy, it needs adequate time to recover. Therefore, you shouldn't do any strenuous activity for the first three months after delivery, and you should wait until your postnatal check-up until you recommence swimming. Giving birth via caesarean will require much more recovery time, and you need to let your body recover fully first. If you had a caesarean, you can still recommence the pelvic-floor stability exercises a day or two after giving birth, but you should wait until your postnatal check-up before recommencing your exercise routine, and you should start with low-impact activities such as walking or bike riding. Pushing your child in their pram around the neighbourhood is a great place to start.

Exercising while breastfeeding

Breastfeeding can make it a little challenging to exercise, not only due to exhaustion from the regular feeding program throughout the night, but also due to some side effects that you may experience from breastfeeding itself (for example, tender breasts and sore, cracked nipples). Many of my patients talk of the struggles when it comes to fatigue after their child is born and often the last thing they want to do is run around the park. But, despite how tired you feel, prioritising exercise will help you not only physically but also mentally, and you will feel more energetic for doing it. It will also help you bounce back quickly to your pre-pregnancy, naturally optimum weight.

Some of the most practical workouts post-pregnancy involve pushing the pram around the neighbourhood and incorporating hills in your route. The best time to do this is between feeds, preferably straight after a feed to reduce the weight of your breasts

(as they do fill up between feeds) and to avoid your child screaming from hunger while you're out. It's also a good idea to provide
extra protection for your nipples because the added friction from
salty sweat running over sore and cracked nipples can be enough to
deter you from vigorous exercise altogether. A breastfeeding sports
bra might also come in handy.

Exercise as a medicine

Physical activity activates the brain's pleasure circuit. Exercise
boosts serotonin levels, consequently improving your mood and
social functioning. Better still, it will prevent impulsive food
choices and it's one of the best forms of stress management, which
is why it's great to ensure your whole family has an active lifestyle.
And if you can get your exercise routine into gear, your pregnancy
and post-pregnancy experience should be easier.

Staying motivated to exercise during and after pregnancy can
be hard, especially when you're sleep deprived and in continual
discomfort, or busy raising your other child or children, so this
can be a good time to mix up where you are exercising. I'm refer-
ring to the physical locations themselves – the streets you are
walking on, the ovals you are training at and the people you
are exercising with. Every time you exercise somewhere different,
you gain a new energy boost that you didn't know existed. This is
due to not only the location itself but also the excitement of going
somewhere new. It's the same reasoning behind offering your
child a range of different experiences when it comes to physical
activity. Every location offers something that the previous place
didn't, and this is the stimulus that you need to stay motivated
and committed to a long-term exercise plan during pregnancy,
after pregnancy and beyond.

CHAPTER 6

SCREEN TIME SHOWDOWN

Of all the parenting challenges the modern world throws up, one of the most contentious and problematic is what to do about screen time. For those of us who have children over the age of one, you will know exactly what I'm talking about – developing and consistently enforcing a set of rules around your child's access to screens is a relentless battle. Smartphones, iPads, laptops and televisions all have an impact on the brain that is linked to our reward system, specifically our endorphins, which make screens highly addictive and affect attention span. This combination means a child will feel a strong urge to interact with 'their' screen while also being unable to concentrate when they don't have it. Children who are addicted to screens often act out when they are denied. It is a continual downward spiral.

Beyond behavioural challenges, too much screen time is proven to cause physical changes to a child's brain. The outer layer of the brain – the cortex – is responsible for complex brain functions, such as controlling language and processing information. The formation of the cortex begins at around 18 days of gestation, but it undergoes critical development during adolescence and continues to develop and mature throughout your twenties. What I'm saying is, when it comes to your child's health, it's never too late to put down the screens, because excessive screen time can affect the growth of the brain, resulting in a thinner cortex. Data for this comes from the largest long-term study of brain development and child health conducted in the United States – the Adolescent Brain Cognitive Development Study. The research shows that those who use screens more often, specifically for non-school related use – and this includes TV, movies, videos, video games, texting, social media and video chat – have poorer sleep health, worse mental health, increased risk of attention deficit hyperactivity disorder (ADHD) and lower grades in school.

The impact of screens stretches beyond the impact on your child's brain. Screen use displaces time that could be spent being physically active. Research also shows that the long-term effects of excessive screen time – defined as upwards of 120 minutes a day – during the first 2000 days of a child's life are linked with long-term weight and health problems. You may have heard the phrase 'sitting is the new smoking' but here's a new one: 'screen time is the new junk food'. The total saturation of screens – mobile phone in the pocket, laptop while working from home, television on in the background – have created a new minefield for parents who have no real playbook to help them navigate this very 21st century issue. The culmination of this is all too often conflict in the family home.

When it comes to what you should allow, the general consensus from governing guidelines is that screen time is not recommended at all for children less than two years of age. For two- to five-year-olds, they should not be using them for more than one hour per day, and by the time they start school, their recreational screen time should be no more than two hours per day.

The proliferation of screens has been beneficial on many fronts but presents new challenges when it comes to our health. You might be wondering what screens have to do with food choices, but the omnipresence of screens means it is vital to delve into this topic. Understanding the impacts of screen time is just as important for your child's lifelong health as food choices and physical inactivity. This brings us to the sixth principle – *screen time showdown*. Having told you the scary side of screen time, I'm now going to give you real-life solutions that will deliver success, if you as the parent commit long term.

Monkey see, monkey do

If you accept that screen time has the potential for long-term detrimental health outcomes for your child, then the first thing you must do is set up the process for how you engage with and absorb your own screen activity. As with the other five principles of this lifestyle plan, it's a whole family approach. This cannot be sugar coated; the discipline starts with you. This means no more dinners in front of the TV, and the TV should not be the first thing that is switched on when you get home. It means no more scrolling on your phone when you are cooking dinner, or at the dinner table, or watching your child in the bath or even during playtime. Put down that phone. Little kids are particularly malleable when it comes to role modelling, but both small children and older kids benefit when you put down your phone and fully engage with them.

One of the unfortunate side effects of being a parent is the underlying fear and anxiety that something bad will happen to your child. Parents often tell me that they always keep their phone on them just in case there is an emergency with their child. While this may be an acceptable reason if you are away from your child and out of the home, it is not needed when you're with them in the home.

Set a rule for yourself that carves out moments in the day where your phone is left in another room. You must leave it there for a set amount of time, and do not break that rule. For example, if you've been at work all day, as soon as you walk in the door, set the phone aside in your bedroom, out of sight, and give your child your full attention until they've gone to bed. Another good option is to put your phone in a drawer while you're playing with your child.

Fight technology with technology

Addiction to technology is a big part of the problem. The good news is that while technology in this instance is the cause of the problem, it can also be the solution. With smartphones, for example, you can change the settings to remotely monitor and manage your child's usage, set screen time limits, and even lock their phone if the limits are exceeded. If that all seems too complicated, there are other solutions too. Certain apps allow a parent on a 'master device', that is, their smartphone or laptop, to shut down nominated apps on their child's device. This can be scheduled or in the moment. By doing it this way, you, the parent, don't have to physically remove the device, which we know leads to so much struggle. You can discreetly, from anywhere, shut down the games, YouTube, TikTok, Snapchat or whatever app is consuming your child's attention. There is a wealth of choice when it comes to parental control apps for your phone. Investigate and adopt the parental control app that you prefer.

You can also have rules like no screens in the bedroom, no mobile phone after a certain time of day or before homework is completed – or go old school and turn off the Wi-Fi. This works well if you have young children, but by the time they are teenagers, it can be the source of a lot of conflict in the house. Talk to them about why you are introducing this rule, or better still, create a plan together so they feel in control of their choices.

No blue light after twilight

The screens of electronic devices such as smartphones, tablets, computers and televisions emit what is known as blue light. This has a reductive effect on melatonin, a hormone designed to tell us to sleep. In turn, this disrupts our natural sleep cycles, resulting in poor sleep health. When you use these devices at night, they are telling your brain it is daytime and not time to close your eyes and get some much-needed rest. Think of blue light from screens working in the brain like a sunrise (which is also high in blue light) triggering you to wake up – not what you want before bed. The human brain needs at least two hours of no screen time before falling asleep so it can recover from and wind down after a day full of blue light.

Removing screens for two hours before bedtime is important for two reasons. Firstly, it allows you and your child to fall asleep faster by decreasing sleep latency – the amount of time it takes to fall to sleep. This ensures you get the deep and restful sleep that mostly occurs during the first half of the night. Secondly, it ensures you get better quality sleep and more of it. Research has shown that anything less than seven hours of sleep disrupts our appetite hormones. The result of this is an increased desire to eat, which leads to an increased level of impulsive behaviour linked to food choices. The impulse is usually to reach for sugar, fats and salts, for immediate gratification. If you miss a few hours of sleep, the next day you may end up heading to the vending machine for a chocolate bar or the corner store for some chips, instead of having a nutritious homemade snack. But it's not just limited to your food choices; sleep deprivation has a flow-on effect to other aspects of your lifestyle too. Feeling tired all the time means you are also more likely to skip structured physical activity because you don't have the energy to move. Research shows that sleep deprivation impacts children, adolescents and adults in similar ways.

Picture a typical day for many families. Children are watching television until they have a bath before bedtime. When the kids are in bed, parents watch their own television until half an hour before bedtime. The parents then go to bed and continue to scroll on their phones until it's 'lights off' time. This results in delayed sleep latency – you have a hard time falling and staying asleep. It also results in a loss of the precious deep sleep, meaning that you are more prone to emotional responses the following day. Your children also wake up deprived of most of their deep sleep thanks to their late-night television watching, and as a result they are more likely to demand sugary breakfasts and quick-fix screen time before they're taken to school or day care. You, as the parent, on account of being tired yourself, succumb to their demands because you just cannot be bothered with the battle. Does this sound familiar to you? We've all been there. But there is a way out.

Precisely two hours before your child's bedtime, all screens of any variety should be turned off with no room for negotiation. Again, if you have older children, discuss with them the issues associated with excessive screen time, and create a plan together so they feel in control of their choices. Research tells us that the cravings for screens start to diminish as you cut back on screen time, and a new, more positive routine will start to form. But it doesn't happen overnight. As I mentioned in chapter 2, it can take on average 66 days for an old habit to go and a new one to form. Put in place the same rule for yourself and pick up a book while you leave your phone charging in the kitchen. This also means removing all screens from the bedroom, including televisions, tablets and computers. Your, and your child's, bedroom should be a place of sanctuary, not work or screen-based entertainment.

To go one step further, you can replace full spectrum light bulbs with warm white bulbs or dimmers to further enhance the sleeping environment and minimise all blue light emission. Decreasing your exposure to blue light in the evening is an important way to help the body naturally prepare for sleep and get quality rest.

How much sleep should your child get?

Your child's sleep patterns will change significantly during their first 12 months. Newborns up to 3 months sleep on and off during the day and night (a total of 15 to 18 hours of sleep over 24 hours). From 3 to 6 months, they start developing a night and day sleep schedule, with a pattern of 90 to 120 minutes sleep, three times a day, and a long sleep during the night that is broken up by several feeds, decreasing as they age (a total of 12 to 15 hours of sleep over 24 hours). As they develop from 6 to 12 months, more of their sleep happens at night, but they will continue to have a couple of daytime naps. Most children will learn to sleep through the night from 12 months (and some much earlier), but it is common for them to wake a couple of times. Just like us, it can take a while for them to wind down before bed, so develop a healthy, consistent bedtime routine with your child. For example, have a bath after dinner, play some gentle music, tell them a story or read a book together. Much like breastfeeding, don't be scared to seek professional help with sleep training, if you are struggling.

The amount of sleep a child requires decreases as they age. From 1 to 2 years, they will need a total of 11 to 14 hours of sleep (10 to 12 hours of sleep at night and 1 to 2 hours during the day). The daytime nap tapers off around 2 to 3 years of age. Children 3 to 4 years of age need 10 to 13 hours of sleep, while for primary school children it's 9 to 11 hours, and for teenagers, 8 to 10 hours.

How much sleep should you get?

Sleep is a big challenge, particularly when you are pregnant or have small children. You must aim to get a minimum of seven hours of sleep per night for your own health. I can hear you saying, 'I don't have time for that' or 'I've never been able to sleep' or 'My children keep me up and I only ever get four hours sleep a night' or 'My partner keeps me awake with their snoring'. If any of these reflect your situation, changes need to be made to take ownership of your health.

The evenings are an exceptionally challenging time for families. We often find ourselves craving an emotional high or wanting something enjoyable to counter a stressful day of running around. After getting the children to bed, we make our way to the couch and unwind with some TV. We combat the stress of the day by reaching for food that makes us feel good – to give us that high. Known as comfort or emotional eating, this happens day after day, and it is quite challenging to control.

The first thing you need to do is fix your food environment. If the block of chocolate is in the cupboard, you're more likely to eat it. It's less tempting when it's not in the home, and this will help guide you towards healthier food choices. If your partner, wife or husband is the one to blame (that is, they are bringing chocolate or wine into the house or having it in front of you every evening), you need to discuss the situation so you are both aligned with your family goals. Better still, get them to read this book.

The second thing you need to change is your evening routine. It's likely you're exhausted from raising one child or multiple children, and from the demands of modern life. Instead of unwinding with your phone or TV after dinner, try brushing your teeth first. You're less likely to look for comfort food if your teeth are already clean. Then relax by working on a hobby, doing some housework, or reading a book. Anything to keep you occupied and away from screens, and less likely to reach for those comfort foods. You will only break an old habit if you replace it with a new one. If you just don't feel like doing anything at all, this is fine too. In many instances, especially if you're a busy mum, dad or guardian, the last thing you want to do at the end of the day is more work. After all, you've spent your entire day looking after your children or working while they were at school. But you still need to have a plan in place to prevent comfort eating and excessive screen time. It might mean treating yourself to a bubble bath with some soothing music and candles. You could also try going for a walk around the block, talking to your partner or doing yoga or meditation. Meditation is a training technique that anyone can do to bring you back into the present moment and to guide your thoughts in a more constructive direction. Simply find a quiet place to sit – either on the floor cross-legged or on a comfortable chair with your feet on the ground, and listen to your breathing. Take deep breaths, in and out, and do this for a few minutes, building it up over time to 10 minutes a day.

If you are suffering from chronic sleep deprivation, it's important to change your routine and go to bed earlier. Set yourself a goal of getting into bed at the same time each day and waking up at the same time every morning. This way you are giving your body the best chance of getting the rest it needs. When it comes to snoring, if you or your partner snore, see your doctor. Weight loss can help with this, but it may also be due to a condition known as sleep apnoea, in which case you may need treatment to improve your sleep quality. Even if you must sleep in separate rooms for a short period of time, it's essential to get your health under control.

The importance of bed quality

Sleep is one of the most important aspects of your and your child's health, so don't be scared to spend some money on it if you can.

It is much more important to spend your money on a good-quality mattress than on a commodity you barely use and often pay more for. We spend approximately one-third of our day in bed – this is much more time than we would spend commuting in our car, for example. So, as soon as you have saved up enough money, invest in some good-quality beds and pillows for you and your children.

Caffeine and alcohol intake

Caffeine is a stimulant (found in chocolate, cocoa, coffee and tea) and should not be consumed within four to six hours of bed. So, if you go to bed at 10 p.m., that means no caffeine after 4 p.m. And be aware that green tea and kombucha tea are not caffeine free. The only tea that is caffeine free is herbal tea, which is based on the herbal infusion from the leaves of the tree.

With respect to alcohol, while it might send you to sleep quickly, you will have a hard time staying asleep and you will wake up feeling tired the next day. If you choose to drink, keep it to one self-pour drink per day (which equates closer to two standard drinks). You should also work towards a minimum of two alcohol-free days per week. Alcohol can still be part of a healthy lifestyle (unless you are pregnant or breastfeeding), but it will affect your sleep quality if you have too much, and it will make it challenging to hit your weight-loss goals if you are consuming more than one standard drink per day.

Pregnancy and sleep

When it comes to pregnancy, there are several sleep problems that you might experience. A common grievance is insomnia; many pregnant women struggle to fall asleep or stay asleep due to lower back pain, breast pain, pelvic girdle pain, nausea, baby movements or due to stress and anxiety about labour and motherhood. Other problems include reflux (heartburn), restless legs (unpleasant feeling in the legs), sleep apnoea (interrupted breathing during sleep) and frequent night-time urination. However, some of these tips may help:

- Exercise every day.
- Read or write in bed instead of forcing yourself to sleep.
- Take a lukewarm bath before bed.
- Avoid eating too much spicy or fried food, particularly before bed.
- Ask your doctor about potential medication for heartburn.
- Make your doctor aware of your snoring habit so they can determine whether you should be screened for sleep apnoea. The same applies to your partner too.
- Drink most of your fluid intake at the start of the day and taper off from 4 p.m. onwards.
- Add a dim light to the bathroom to avoid you having to turn on the light each time you wake during the night.

Children and sleep deprivation

Sleep deprivation is no joke for new mums and dads. It can also be challenging for those with older children or teens. Just when you manage to get on top of all the sleep issues caused during pregnancy, new problems can arise, and therefore most women need to pay close attention to their sleep after they give birth. Each person will experience different challenges but the most common relate to frequency of the feeding schedule, difficulties getting your child to fall asleep and developmental challenges such as teething and growth spurts. Before allowing your sleep deprivation to hit rock bottom, you should implement the following tips:

1. Change your usual routine. You may think that turning on the TV after your child goes to sleep is your time to unwind and relax, but it's going to do more harm than good. Not only will it increase your chance of comfort eating, but it's also going to see you getting less rest. You need to adjust your sleep routine after your child is born and ensure you go to bed at the same time each night, and much earlier than you are used to, in order to compensate for the night-time waking up that is unavoidable for at least the first few months.

2. Seek professional help and implement sleep training. There are various methods and I'm not here to add to the collection of sleep training books, but it's something you should consider well before problems arise, often as early as four months of age.

3. Sleep when your child sleeps. There is no harm in lying down when your child does if you can. While it's not always possible to sleep, even a 20-minute nap can help.

4. If you have friends and family nearby who want to help, accept their offers. It might give you that little bit of assistance you need to ensure extra rest.

5. Consider pumping or using formula. If you have a partner or someone who can help, pump some breastmilk ahead of time, so they can take control of one of the feeding shifts. You can also try using formula for specific feeds.

6. Consider that older children and teenagers are often most communicative before bedtime. Allowing them ample opportunity and plenty of attention during and after the evening meal can help account for this and prevent the situation where you go to bed later than expected.

CHAPTER 7

COMMONLY ASKED QUESTIONS

When it comes to their family's health, there are a few questions parents often ask me. This section is designed to be a comprehensive catalogue of the common stumbling blocks when first starting out, a chapter you can turn to as needed. However, if you have a question that isn't covered here, I encourage you to get in touch through my website, feedingfussykids.com.

Is this plan for all families?

I have received countless enquiries about whether this whole family approach is a lifestyle plan that can be followed by people of different ethnicities or with different eating patterns. The answer is yes, absolutely yes! The whole family approach can be followed by anyone. This plan is an adaptive approach that can be tailored to suit your lifestyle and your individual circumstances. If your family is vegetarian, take the meat out and supplement with a different source of protein. If someone is allergic to shellfish, try a tofu recipe instead. If there's a coeliac in your family, substitute bread and other gluten sources with gluten-free wholegrain carbohydrates.

As long as you follow the six principles outlined in this book, you can make whatever adjustments you and your family need.

Can this plan be followed by someone with diabetes and polycystic ovary syndrome (PCOS)?

Yes, this whole family approach is most certainly suitable for people with diabetes – both type 1 and type 2, and gestational diabetes (diabetes during pregnancy) – and women with PCOS. If you have type 2 diabetes, making changes to your health as outlined in this lifestyle plan will help prevent the disease from progressing further, and in some instances, it may help you reverse the disease. It is also suitable for those with insulin resistance or pre-diabetes (the stage before type 2 diabetes), because these lifestyle changes will help your body work properly again and improve your overall health.

PCOS is a common hormonal disorder that affects a woman's ovaries during her childbearing years. It can cause a variety of uncomfortable and painful symptoms, including irregular periods, acne and fertility problems. If you or someone in your family has PCOS, lifestyle changes and healthy weight management can help manage the symptoms and regulate ovulation and periods.

Is this plan suitable for people with food intolerances?

Yes, because this whole family approach is entirely adaptable. If there is a recipe that includes milk, for instance, and someone in your family is lactose intolerant, you can substitute it with a lactose-free alternative, such as lactose-free milk. Similarly, if someone in your family has coeliac disease, you can eliminate ingredients containing gluten and find a gluten-free replacement, such as those mentioned in this book.

Is this plan suitable for families following a vegan or vegetarian eating plan?

Yes, most certainly. Again, simply substitute any meat or animal products with suitable alternatives. For example, replace meat with tofu, or chicken with beans. Refer to chapter 3 for a key list of nutrients to be mindful of when following a vegan diet.

Can I substitute the recipes in this book with my own favourites?

Yes, absolutely. The recipes in Part 2 are simply a guide. This book is not intended to be a cookbook but rather to give you some good ideas for healthy meals you can make, how easy it can be to cook using just a few ingredients, and to show you which nutritious ingredients you should use as the foundations for all recipes. You can include any of your favourite recipes into your family's weekly food plan; you may just have to make some alterations to them to ensure they uphold the core principles of this plan. Remember the following:

- Cook with raw ingredients.
- Use canola or olive oil only (preferably extra virgin or cold-pressed varieties).
- Include plenty of vegetables or leafy greens with each recipe (especially with pasta-based meals).
- Ensure there is a source of fat, protein and wholegrain carbohydrate with each recipe so the daily meal plan is nutritionally balanced and includes all the core food groups.

Is sugar bad for my child?

Since the 'sugar free' and 'I Quit Sugar' movements became popular, there has been much confusion about what constitutes a sugar and the difference between various types of sugars. Added sugars and naturally occurring sugars are not the same thing. Many foods contain naturally occurring sugars (for example, fruit and dairy), and these foods are still good for us. They are excellent sources of nutrition and important for your child's long-term health. Do not let someone convince you that just because a food contains sugar, it is automatically bad for you. They are wrong. Naturally occurring sugars, such as glucose, fructose, sucrose, lactose and maltose are good for us because they are contained in foods that are wholesome and nutritious.

Added sugars are the 'bad' sugars, which are better to avoid. You will find them predominantly in packaged food products, such as muesli bars, or in refined carbs such as pastries, confectionary and sweets. As a rule of thumb, food in its natural form may contain sugars that are naturally occurring and good for us, and food coming out of a packet may contain added sugars that are bad for us. As has been reiterated throughout this book, there is no need to restrict any foods in their naturally occurring form.

Does sugar cause diabetes?

Sugar in foods does *not* cause diabetes. Type 1 diabetes is an autoimmune disease (there is no cure, and it can't be prevented) and type 2 diabetes is typically caused by carrying excess body weight, which consequently stops the body working as efficiently as it should. Gestational diabetes is a type of diabetes developed during pregnancy (closely aligned with type 2 diabetes) and typically goes away following the birth of your child. However, if you do develop it, it is vital to manage it by following the principles of this plan, in conjunction with your diabetes care team, to reduce your risk of pregnancy complications and the risk to your newborn (these risks can include a large birth weight, miscarriage or stillbirth). This will also help to reduce the risk of elevated blood glucose and type 2 diabetes after birth.

Foods that contain *added* sugar and fat, such as pastries, chocolates, ice cream or anything that is processed and coming out of a packet, are high in energy. If you regularly include a high intake of these foods in your diet, it is likely you are eating too many calories and will put on unnecessary weight, which may put you on track to develop type 2 diabetes. However, sugar itself does not cause diabetes.

Sugar is a perplexing field to navigate when wading through the supermarket; there are more than 40 names for sugar. The most common ingredients to watch out for when looking for added sugars on labels include:

- brown sugar
- corn syrup
- fruit juice concentrate
- glucose solids
- high-fructose corn syrup
- invert sugar
- malt sugar
- molasses
- raw sugar
- sugar
- sugar molecules ending in 'ose' (for example, dextrose, glucose, sucrose, maltose, fructose).

Should fruit be avoided because it contains sugar?

Yes, fruit does contain sugar but as I've outlined throughout this book, these are naturally occurring sugars. They are nature's treats and should form part of you and your child's daily eating plan. Do not worry about how much fruit your child is eating. They can eat as much whole fruit as they like, as long as it's not juiced or dried. Juicing means most of the goodness (the fibre) gets left behind in the juicer, and dried fruit has had the water stripped out of it, so it's very easy to overconsume. Fruit or other foods containing naturally occurring sugars do not cause diabetes or weight gain. You can give your child all fruits on this plan (yes, even bananas!).

If I buy skim or low-fat milk, will it contain added sugar?

Skim, no-fat or low-fat milk does not contain added sugar. The only difference between full-fat and low-fat or skim alternatives is that the fat has literally been skimmed off the top of the milk. Skim or low-fat milk will have the same protein and calcium as regular milk, just without the fat. Some milks do contain added sugar, though, such as almond milk, oat milk and other dairy alternatives. Always read the label carefully.

Which milk is best?

Breastmilk or formula is the only milk you should give your child up until 12 months of age. However, it's important to point out that, although a point of contention in Australia, the World Health Organisation has updated its guidelines to say full-fat animal milk can be given to non-breastfed or mixed-fed babies between 6 and 12 months as an alternative to formula.

After your child turns one, you can substitute breastmilk or formula for cow's milk. Cow's milk is the richest source of calcium, protein and iodine, but not all children can tolerate it. Your child might be dairy-intolerant or lactose-intolerant. If you are looking for a dairy-free and lactose-free alternative to cow's milk, calcium-fortified soy milk is the next best option from a nutritional perspective. If you are looking for a lactose-free milk alternative to regular cow's milk, opt for lactose-free milk, which you will find in both the fresh milk section and long-life shelves in the supermarket. If your child is intolerant to both soy and dairy (which they often outgrow by the age of three to five years), the next best alternative is calcium-fortified oat milk, but make sure to check the protein content as it can vary between brands. Plant-based alternatives such as rice milk and almond milk are low in protein and are better left on the shelves. Tune into my podcast with Dr Karl on 'white drink scams' for more information, which you can find at the University of Sydney's 'Shirtloads of Science' page (shirtloadsofscience.libsyn.com/sos-114-nf-alt-milk).

Which yoghurt should I give my child?

You do need to be a little careful when it comes to yoghurt. No-fat or low-fat yoghurt may contain added sugar to make up for the loss of flavour incurred by removing the fat. You can buy no-fat and low-fat yoghurt without added sugar, or better still, you can opt for plain, natural yoghurt and add your own sweetness with fruit or honey.

Is it okay to give my child full-fat dairy?

Yes, it is. And you should give them full-fat varieties at least until they are two years of age. In fact, you don't need to be buying no-fat or low-fat dairy products at all, the full-fat variety is perfectly fine. Children need a lot of calcium, and the best form of calcium is dairy.

Are products such as Weet-Bix and All-Bran cereal okay to give my child?

Despite coming out of a packet, some breakfast cereal products are obviously better than others – these include the ones that are largely wholegrain-wheat based, such as Weet-Bix and All-Bran. However, it is important to bear in mind that such packaged products will also contain other added ingredients such as salt and added sugar, and there are many more suitable breakfast options such as eggs, oats, avocado on wholegrain toast, or fruit and yoghurt. Try to stay clear of all processed cereal products; it's just as easy to make something much healthier and more nutritious from scratch.

Can my child eat any type of nuts and seeds?

Yes, providing they don't have a nut allergy. You should introduce nuts into your child's diet as early as possible (from four to six months) and in the form of 100 per cent nut spreads. Current guidelines advise not giving your child whole nuts until they are five years old due to the risk of choking. All nuts are good. Choose dry-roasted nuts or those in their natural form, without added oil or salt.

Are activated almonds better for my child than normal almonds?

No! 'Activation' does not improve the digestibility and nutrition of the nut, despite all the clever marketing surrounding it.

Can my child have wholegrain carbs if they are diagnosed with coeliac disease?

Yes, definitely. If your child is diagnosed with coeliac disease, you need to avoid grains containing gluten, such as wheat, rye and barley. Suitable gluten-free whole grains that are also rich in fibre include rice, quinoa, millet and amaranth, and you should include plenty of them in your child's diet (see some suggestions of other suitable whole grains in chapter 3). There are also many foods that are naturally free of gluten – fruits, vegetables, dairy, meat, fish, nuts and eggs, to name a few. To get tested for coeliac disease, your GP may send your child for a blood test in the first instance, but to confirm the diagnosis they will need to send them for an endoscopy – a specialised test where they check the lining of your child's intestine to see if it is functioning properly.

Does soda water contain sugar and can my child drink it instead of water?

Commercially bought soda water does not contain sugar, but it does contain sodium, so your child shouldn't be drinking it as their primary source of fluid. It should be a treat only. Even mineral or sparkling water can contain sodium, depending on the brand, so be sure to check what you're buying if it's a regular item in your household. And for those who drink tonic water, this does contain sugar, so try to stick to the 'diet' option if you don't forgo it entirely. Remember, it's a treat too. Make sure to listen to my episode 'Do soft drinks shorten your life?' on the *9 Minutes to Better Health* podcast.

How do I know how much to eat?

We all need guidance, but relying on calorie-controlled meal plans is not healthy or sustainable. You must learn how much to eat at each meal by listening to your body's appetite signals and by ensuring that you eat a lot at the start of the day and very little towards the end of the day. For most, this will mean completely switching around the structure of your current food intake. If you're having oats for breakfast, load up your bowl, because breakfast is the most important meal of the day and should be the biggest (but you can split it up into two smaller breakfasts if that works better for you – perhaps one before work and one when you arrive at work). If you can't get through the whole portion or feel uncomfortably full at the end of the meal, you have eaten too much, and you need to reduce the quantity the next day until you strike the right balance. Everyone's needs are different. Also, men will usually need more food than women (sometimes one and a half times the intake) because they have a larger body mass. During pregnancy, your appetite will increase too to compensate for the child you are growing.

The same rule applies to dinner. If a recipe specifies how many serves it makes, it is just a guide. Portions can vary enormously between you and your child, and your normal appetite versus your appetite during pregnancy or when you are breastfeeding. You might also want to make an appropriate amount to factor in leftovers for the next day's lunch. And it depends on which meal you cook the recipe for, because it is important to serve up a larger portion at lunch than what you would at dinner.

As a general rule of thumb, when you are first starting out on this plan, and to give you a guide, your breakfast portion size will be equivalent to three handprints (measured from the top of your middle finger to the base of your palm and the same thickness of your palm) or three closed fists, your lunch will be approximately two times your handprint or two times your closed fist, and your evening meal will be approximately one handprint or one closed fist. (Remember, these guides exclude vegetables, so you can load up your plate with as many vegetables and salad as you like at each meal.) Your food requirements will increase during pregnancy (particularly during the third trimester) and when breastfeeding – up to one and a third times the amount of food you typically eat. This is perfectly normal and encouraged.

Another great tool to use is the appetite scale provided on page 26. This may be particularly helpful when you are first starting on this plan; you can continually assess how hungry you are before and after each meal. You need to record this before and after each meal in a food journal to fine-tune your portions over time.

In summary, there are no exact portion sizes that you need to focus on for you or your family. But every meal must be balanced. For you, half the meal should be vegetables or salad, with a quarter being a wholegrain carbohydrate source, such as a piece of bread or a serve of rice, and a quarter being your protein source such as meat, fish or lentils. For your child, one-third of the meal should be vegetables or salad, one-third a wholegrain carbohydrate source such as a piece of bread or serve of rice, and one-third a protein source such as meat, fish or lentils.

How do I meet my nutritional requirements when struggling with morning sickness?

Morning sickness is common during pregnancy, usually in the first trimester, and mostly due to changing levels of pregnancy hormones. It's vital to keep well hydrated, even if you can only manage small, frequent sips of fluid. Soups are another great way of keeping up your fluid intake to prevent dehydration while also getting extra nutrients. During this time, it is more appropriate to eat smaller, more regular meals. It is also advised to avoid any foods whose smells make your nausea worse, and you may need to focus on including blander food in your diet until the morning sickness eases.

I never wake up hungry. What should I do?

It takes time for your hunger cues to change, and if you have been doing the same thing for years or decades – that is, skipping breakfast because you didn't feel hungry – your body's signals will not change overnight. Coffee can also mask your appetite, so make sure to eat something with your morning coffee. If you are eating late at night or overeating in the evening, you also need to make some changes to ensure you start waking up hungrier.

If you have changed your meal structure to ensure you are eating most of your food at the start of the day and less at the end of the day, you are well on the way to success and you will start to wake up feeling hungrier. Just give it time! This change won't happen overnight.

How much should I eat during pregnancy?

Your appetite will increase during the second and particularly the third trimester of pregnancy. This is normal; welcome this increase in appetite. It may mean you're eating one and a third times the quantity of food you typically eat (this is fine and encouraged). You are growing another person, and they are dependent on your good nutrition to grow and develop. Always remember to *reach for nature first* and whenever you have cravings for junk food, think about your health and that of your baby. Listen to your body's appetite signalling and feed it the fuel it needs. If you're still hungry after eating, have some more.

How much should I eat while breastfeeding?

Much like during pregnancy, your appetite will increase when breastfeeding and will only start to decrease when your baby starts to eat solids. Making breastmilk burns a lot of calories, and you need extra food to meet these requirements. Again, just like when you're pregnant, you may be eating one and a third times the amount of food you normally do, and this is perfectly fine. You need to listen to what your body is telling you – if you're hungry, you need to eat. Remember, the breastmilk you are producing is your baby's only fuel source and the nutrition you take in will influence their food preferences later in life. Eat according to the principles of this plan and, importantly, focus on including a rich variety of foods in your diet.

Is it bad to eat carbs for dinner when pregnant?

No; you should eat carbs with every meal. Choose wholegrain types to ensure every meal is balanced and to help you feel fuller for longer. There is no research to suggest that eating carbs at night makes you put on weight.

Should I take supplements during pregnancy? If so, which ones?

It is best to consult with your general practitioner before attempting to fall pregnant. There are three vitamins and nutrients that you should take during pregnancy as a supplement. This is because your body has different requirements during pregnancy and you're unlikely to get enough from the foods you eat, or from sunshine.

Make sure to take a pregnancy-specific supplement each day that contains:

- Folic acid: 500 micrograms (may also be written as 0.5 milligrams)
- Iodine: 150 micrograms
- Vitamin D: 400 international units (may also be written as 10 micrograms).

Only take a multivitamin designed for pregnancy, because other supplements may contain vitamins that are harmful at high doses during pregnancy (for example, vitamin A/retinol).

Folate, or folic acid, is a vitamin that helps reduce the risk of certain birth defects such as spina bifida. Start taking folate when planning your pregnancy and continue for the first three months of pregnancy. If there is a family history of cleft lip, spinal problems, you are taking an anti-epilepsy medication or you have type 1 or type 2 diabetes, this dose may need to be greater. It is best to consult with your doctor.

Iodine is a nutrient that is important for your baby's brain development. It's found in many foods such as fish, dairy and iodised salt, but to make sure you meet your requirement take a supplement that contains at least 150 micrograms of iodine. You should avoid seaweed tablets as the iodine dose can be too high.

Vitamin D is important for the development of your baby's bones and teeth. It is mostly made in the skin by the action of sunlight, but a small amount can come from foods such as oily fish and egg yolks. Low levels can cause muscle weakness and pain in women, and skeletal problems (called rickets) in newborns. If you have low levels of vitamin D, you will need to take an even higher dose than the recommended 400 international units (IU) per day during pregnancy to correct the deficiency. This need is determined by a blood test through your doctor.

Iron, calcium, omega-3 and vitamin B12 supplements may also be required during pregnancy, but only in consultation with your doctor.

Iron

Iron is needed to make red blood cells that carry oxygen around the body. During pregnancy you need more iron because the volume of your blood increases and your baby's blood is also developing. It is important for pregnant women to eat iron-rich foods every day. Animal sources of iron (for example, red meat) are readily absorbed by the body. Iron from plant sources is not absorbed as easily, but absorption is helped when these foods are eaten together with foods that contain vitamin C (such as oranges). Symptoms of low iron include tiredness and lack of energy. A deficiency can be detected through an iron-studies blood test by your doctor, which you should do before taking any supplements.

Calcium

Calcium is important for bone health and preventing osteoporosis, also known as brittle bones. Dairy foods are the richest source of calcium and are of the highest bioavailability, meaning there is a higher absorption rate of calcium from the food. You need two to three serves of calcium-rich foods each day. If you don't eat dairy or other calcium-fortified milks (such as soy), talk to your doctor about whether you need a calcium supplement.

Omega-3

Omega-3 fatty acids are needed for healthy brain, nerve and eye development in your baby. They also help reduce inflammation in your body. Eating foods rich in omega-3 fatty acids, such as fish, or plant-based sources such as nuts and seeds will help meet you and your baby's needs. Aim to include fish in your diet three times per week and a handful of nuts each day. If you don't eat fish, you'll probably need a fish-oil supplement, and you need to be taking 3000 milligrams per day to get the benefit (usually 3 to 6 tablets per day depending on the strength of the supplements you buy). Make sure to store them in the fridge to prevent them oxidising.

Vitamin B12

Vitamin B12 is required for the formation of red blood cells as well as a healthy brain and nervous system. It is only found in animal products. It is *not* found in plant sources of food and therefore it is vital to choose B12-fortified foods such as breakfast cereals and soy products – soy milk, tofu and miso. Even with an increased intake of B12 fortified foods, it will be difficult to achieve an adequate intake. If you are vegan, you will need a vitamin B12 supplement. Vitamin B12 levels can be detected by a blood test. Consult with your general practitioner for a subcutaneous injection or an appropriate supplement.

I don't have time to prepare lunch. Can I eat the same thing every day?

Yes, you can. But, easier still, this whole family approach is a lifestyle plan that advocates for people to cook extra food every night so that you always have leftovers for lunch the next day. If this doesn't work for you and you are convinced you will eat the whole damn lot for dinner even after it's packed away in the fridge, yes, you can make the same lunch each day, as long as you focus on the tunnel plan of eating big to small meals throughout the day. If you don't eat enough at the start of the day, you will always be hungry at the end of the day.

Is it okay to have a sandwich for lunch?

Yes, this is a great lunch option for you and your child. If the sandwich incorporates a wholegrain carb, a protein source, a healthy fat source, and plenty of veg or salad, it gets a tick of approval. Despite what some of your friends or colleagues might think (and say), sandwiches are healthy. Let them eat their keto meal or paleo plate of meat – you just need to worry about yourself and stick to the principles of this plan. Good sandwich toppings include egg, lettuce, salmon, chicken, tomato, capsicum, spinach and so on – get creative!

Should our family only be eating 'clean' foods?

The whole concept of 'clean eating' has done nothing except contribute to the ever-growing diet industry; it's a very clever money maker. The reason it grabs people's attention is because it's catchy. Worryingly, it has morphed into a misleading phrase that has led people to think certain fruits and vegetables are bad for them; that carbohydrates are the cause of all things evil; that you should eat gluten-free foods even when you don't have a gluten intolerance; that coconut oil is a miracle food; and that you should obsess about every little ingredient you add to your meals. Don't get caught in the trap; stay focused on what you are setting out to achieve with the principles of this plan and eat wholesome, nutritious foods.

Are superfoods any good?

The term 'superfood' has gained enormous traction and popularity because, after all, it's something we all want – a food that promises to be super healthy, meaning we can eat it and continue with our other unhealthy lifestyle habits. The promise is that all we need to do is add some acai berries, chia seeds, kale, coconut oil or almond milk to our meal. Acai berries, for example, are packed with anti-oxidants, vitamins and minerals, but so too are all berries, so it doesn't matter which ones your child has – and they should be getting a variety. Kale also contains plenty of vitamins, minerals and antioxidants, but you won't get any more superpowers from eating kale than you would from any other vegetable. All vegetables contain varying amounts of vitamins and minerals, and they are all good for your health. As for the plethora of other cleverly marketed superfoods, don't get caught up in the hype – you will get all the benefits they promise from the foods prescribed in this plan, and you will save a lot of money in the process.

Where do I go for further help? Can I get face-to-face consults?

The good news is that you do not need face-to-face contact to succeed with the lifestyle changes and advice prescribed in this book. You will reap the most benefits when you read this book more than once and embrace the principles it outlines, as this will help you unlearn any unhealthy habits and wrong information you may have picked up over the years, as well as helping you avoid passing them on to your child. Remember that the primary goal is health, not weight. Weight loss should never be prescribed to your child.

I have had a long career as a clinical researcher dealing with patients face to face, and now I want to reach as many people as possible through my books and websites. If you do need to lose weight, again the focus needs to be on health, not a number on the scale. Make sure to check out my advice at intervalweightloss.com or find the Interval Weight Loss app at the Apple or Google Play stores.

PART 2

CREATIVE COOKING

This section of the book is intended to provide you with some examples of the types of meals you can cook for – and with – the family. It is not intended to be a cookbook but instead it will give you some ideas for what you can cook, teach how easy it can be to cook healthy, well-rounded meals using just a few ingredients, and show you what ingredients you should use as the foundations for all recipes. All these recipes are easily adapted; if you don't like tofu, use chicken instead. If you don't have a gluten-free sauce on hand, use the regular kind – the gluten-free option isn't healthier, unless you're cooking for a person with coeliac disease, that is. Unlike some prescriptive cookbooks and methodologies, these recipes are based on general health rather than an arbitrary calorie count, so they are very easy to modify. Some of them even have accompanying videos showing how to cook the recipe, found at feedingfussykids.com, or you can access them by scanning the QR codes on the page. I'm not talking about laborious Michelin-star recipes that take hours to prepare. I'm talking about fun and easy recipes that anyone can cook, and, importantly, recipes the whole family can eat.

Cooking is a wonderful and fulfilling aspect of a healthy lifestyle as it encourages us to appreciate the food we eat. Not only will it ensure you are eating better, but it will also save you money. It can be very easy if you stick to just a few ingredients and recipes that don't take all night to cook. Check the shopping list on page 42 to ensure you have all the core staples on hand. Like the recipes themselves, these ingredients are easily adapted – if you don't like basil, or have run out, it's perfectly fine to omit it or replace with another fresh herb, such as parsley. You shouldn't have to spend all afternoon at the supermarket looking for obscure ingredients and all evening in the kitchen cooking. No one has time to do that, least of all time-poor parents. Everyone can learn the basics of cooking – it just takes a little practice. Your children should be part of the cooking experience as it will teach them important life skills and encourage healthy food habits. And you don't need to wait until they're grown up; children as young as three years of age will benefit from getting involved in the kitchen. Try to think of it as an activity rather than a means to an end; it'll make the flour that inevitably gets dropped on the floor and chickpeas strewn over the counter less annoying.

Much the same can be said when catering for the entire family. No one has the time to cook separate meals for different members of the family (and nor should they). Everyone in the family should be eating the same meals, and, whenever possible, they should eat together at the dining table. Many of the recipes in this book can simply be mashed or thrown in the blender so your young child who is just getting introduced to solid foods can also enjoy them. That way you will only find yourself cooking one meal, instead of many!

A recipe gets the tick of approval if it includes unprocessed or raw ingredients, plenty of vegetables (fresh or frozen) or salad, a lean protein source, a wholegrain carbohydrate and a healthy fat, such as extra virgin olive oil. It can be just as easy to cook with raw produce as it is to use pre-made ingredients, which are often expensive and full of additives compared to their whole-food counterparts. But there are times when pre-made foods do play a role, such as pastry or stock – there was once a time when we made stock ourselves in our family home, but those days are over. Some things just aren't practical when juggling all of the demands of modern life. When it comes to shopping, opt for the salt-reduced version of stock and tomato paste instead of the regular varieties. With regards to seasoning with salt and pepper, most of us tend to over-season our food, leading to an excess consumption of salt. To help wean yourself off this dependency, try making these recipes without the usual generous serving of salt you might add, even if it's half what you'd normally include. Eventually, you'll find that your tastebuds change and you'll add less and less salt to your meals. Lastly, with respect to spice, some of the recipes in this book may be a little hot for your child, so either reduce the quantity of spice or leave out the chilli entirely, depending on their level of tolerance.

Even if you have never tried cooking, give it a go. This whole family approach to cooking is designed to be simple and easy to follow, while also making sure you and your child are eating healthy and nutritious meals.

Portion sizes

The serving size listed for each recipe is not gospel; rather, it is provided as a guide. This is deliberate, as I've explained throughout the book. Also, a toddler will eat a lot less than older children or teenagers, so the number of serves you get from a recipe will depend on the age of your children.

Breakfast is the most important meal for the whole family. Your child will dictate when and how much they need to eat across the course of the day. But with respect to you, it is important to monitor your hunger signals so that you can adjust your food intake and portions accordingly. You will need to taper off your food intake throughout the day so that breakfast is the biggest meal, lunch is the next biggest and dinner is the smallest.

To give you a very rough guide, breakfast will be a portion size that is equivalent to three closed hand fists, lunch will be two closed hand fists and dinner will be just one (not including salad and vegetables, which you can eat in unlimited amounts with each meal). Some people will need more; for example, you might need four closed hand fists at breakfast, three at lunch and two at dinner to feel satisfied. And others will need less. It is simply a starting point to help kickstart the process. As long as you are eating most of your food from breakfast through to lunch and dinner is your smallest meal, you are doing well.

If you notice that your hunger is still higher before meals at the end of the day, you have some adjustments to make. Your body's hunger signals won't change overnight, especially if you have been eating in the same way for decades (such as skipping breakfast and eating little throughout the day, only to have your biggest meal in the evening). This takes time to change, but if you do adjust your food structure and intake as outlined in this plan, you will start to wake up hungrier in the morning, and you will feel better for it.

Fresh vegetables and herbs

There's a lot to be said for growing your own vegetables and herbs, and you don't need a big garden to do so. Some of the best veggie gardens I have seen are grown on cleverly configured green walls in small apartments. Having your own veggie garden doesn't require much effort, and just a little maintenance will ensure you have an ongoing supply of fresh produce at your fingertips. As we covered in chapter 4, kids will love helping, even if it's just watering the plants. They will be way more thrilled to eat their own cucumber or tomato than one from the supermarket too. The only exception is if your place doesn't get any sunlight – then you will struggle to grow your own produce and will need to stick to buying from the supermarket, or perhaps consider getting involved in a community garden project.

The core staples of any basic garden may include rosemary, basil, parsley, shallots, coriander and rainbow spinach, or another leafy green such as kale, baby spinach or rocket. Mint is another handy herb to grow as it is good for warding off bugs and flies. Be careful, though, as it behaves like a weed and can take over your entire veggie garden. Coriander can be a challenging herb to grow, but the others will often thrive as long as they have some sunlight, water and good, nutrient-rich soil. Don't buy cheap potting mix as it will only ensure failure; invest in a good-quality vegetable soil. Tomatoes are also a wonderful and easy form of produce to grow, and you will notice they taste much sweeter than any variety you buy from the supermarket.

Picking your own fresh produce is extremely satisfying and, if you grow everything from seeds, extremely cost effective. Think about all those times you've bought expensive fresh herbs from the supermarket, only to use a small quantity and see the rest go to waste. Having your own veggie garden is also a great way to involve your children at mealtimes too. Handing them the responsibility for picking the crops is a way for them to contribute to the family meal.

Visit your local nursery for advice about what you can grow in your home environment and which soil to use. Start small and expand your collection of herbs as you gain understanding about what grows best and at what time of the year. For those who develop a green thumb, the opportunities are endless.

BREAKFAST

STICKY DATE BAKED OATS

A delicious and decadent tasting breakfast recipe, inspired by sticky date pudding.

Serves 2–4

Prep Time: 10 minutes
Cooking Time: 30 minutes

4 Medjool dates, pitted
⅓ cup (80 ml) boiling water
1 cup (90 g) rolled oats
⅔ cup (160 ml) milk
1 small banana
2 teaspoons baking powder
Large pinch of ground cinnamon
2 tablespoons 100% natural almond butter, to serve
2 tablespoons Greek yoghurt, to serve

1. Preheat the oven to 180°C (fan-forced). Place the dates into a small bowl and add the boiling water. Set aside to soak for 5 minutes.
2. Transfer the soaked dates and the soaking liquid to a small blender. Add the rolled oats, milk, banana, baking powder and cinnamon. Blend until well combined.
3. Transfer the batter to a 30 cm × 20 cm (approx.) ovenproof dish. Bake for 25–30 minutes until risen and lightly golden on top. The centre should still be soft and dense, like a sticky date pudding.
4. Scoop into bowls and serve topped with the almond butter and yoghurt. If you are serving to young children, allow to cool completely before serving.

BABY-FRIENDLY BIRCHER

Bircher Muesli is a delicious breakfast that is great for the whole family. If you are making this for yourself or for older children, you can top this with some honey and toasted nuts such as walnuts, and some fresh berries.

Serves 4

Prep Time: 5 minutes + overnight refrigeration

2 pink lady apples
2 cups (180 g) rolled oats
1 cup (280 g) Greek yoghurt
1 cup (250 ml) milk
Sprinkle of ground cinnamon

1. Grate the apples, including the peel, into a medium mixing bowl.
2. If you are preparing this recipe for your baby, place the oats into a blender and pulse until the oats reach the consistency of flour. If you are preparing this recipe for adults or older children, skip this step and leave the rolled oats as they are.
3. Add the oats, yoghurt, milk and cinnamon to the apple and mix well to combine. Cover and place in the fridge to soak overnight.
4. To serve, divide the mixture between 4 bowls. If you are preparing this recipe for small children you could make smaller servings and keep the remainder for one more night in the fridge.

MINI BANANA PANCAKES

These mini pancake bites are a great breakfast or snack option. They don't store very well, so make them fresh and serve right away. You can serve these pancakes on their own, or with some fruit, honey and yoghurt.

Makes about 30

Prep Time: 5 minutes
Cooking Time: 15 minutes

1 egg
⅓ cup (80 ml) milk
½ cup (80 g) wholemeal self-raising flour
Sprinkle of ground cinnamon
Olive oil spray
2 bananas, cut into 1 cm slices

1. Whisk the egg and milk in a mixing bowl until combined. Add the flour and cinnamon and whisk until no lumps remain.
2. Spray a large frying pan with olive oil spray. Heat over medium heat.
3. Working in batches, use a fork to dip the banana pieces into the pancake batter and drain off a little of the excess, then place into the frying pan. Fry for 2 minutes until the mini pancakes start to bubble, then flip over and cook for 1–2 minutes on the other side. Remove from the pan.
4. Continue cooking the mini pancakes in batches until all of the banana slices and pancake batter have been used. Serve warm.

MINI BAKED OAT CUPS

These are great for breakfast (perfect for an on-the-go brekky) or even as a snack. They can be made in advance, so are handy to have in the fridge.

Makes 18

Prep Time: 10 minutes
Cooking Time: 15 minutes

Olive oil spray
2 overripe bananas
1 egg
½ cup (125 ml) milk
2 cups (180 g) rolled oats
Pinch of ground cinnamon
¾ cup (115 g) frozen raspberries, thawed

1. Preheat the oven to 180°C (fan-forced). Lightly grease 18 holes of two 12-hole mini muffin trays with olive oil spray.
2. Place the bananas into a mixing bowl and mash well with a fork. Add the egg and mix into the banana until well combined. Add the milk and rolled oats, and stir until evenly combined. Stir in the cinnamon and raspberries.
3. Use a tablespoon to scoop the oat mixture into the muffin trays. Ensure that the oat mixture fills each muffin hole to the top.
4. Bake for 15 minutes, until the oat cups have risen and are slightly golden on top. Cool in the tray for 5 minutes.
5. Lift the oat cups out and cool completely before serving. Keep in the fridge for up to 3 days, or freeze in an airtight freezer bag for up to 2 weeks.

CRUNCHY GLUTEN-FREE GRANOLA (with video)

This granola is gluten-free and makes a satisfying, delicious and filling breakfast. Serve with milk, a dollop of Greek yoghurt and some seasonal fruit. Feel free to substitute whatever nuts and seeds you already have on hand.

Serves 8

Prep Time: 10 minutes
Cooking Time: 40 minutes

2 cups (40 g) puffed brown rice (see Note)
1 cup (160 g) raw almonds
¼ cup (40 g) pepitas
1 tablespoon hemp seeds
1 tablespoon chia seeds
2 teaspoons ground cinnamon
⅓ cup (80 ml) olive oil
⅓ cup (120 g) honey

1. Preheat the oven to 180°C (fan-forced). Line a large rimmed baking tray with baking paper.
2. Place the puffed rice, almonds, pepitas, hemp seeds, chia seeds and cinnamon into a large mixing bowl. Stir to combine.
3. Pour in the olive oil and honey. Stir well to ensure everything is combined and coated. Transfer to the prepared tray and spread out evenly.
4. Bake for 35–40 minutes, taking out to stir every 15 minutes, until crisp and golden. Keep an eye on it as it can brown very quickly.
5. Set aside to cool completely, then transfer to an airtight jar. Keep for up to 1 month in the pantry.

Note: You can find puffed brown rice at health food or bulk food stores.

VEGAN BANANA PANCAKES (with video)

These vegan pancakes are quick and easy to make for a wholesome breakfast. Why not experiment with different flavour combinations – for example you could swap out the cinnamon for lemon zest and frozen blueberries. Serve with a generous drizzle of nut butter for some extra protein.

Serves 4

Prep Time: 10 minutes
Cooking Time: 15 minutes

2 cups (180 g) rolled oats
2 overripe bananas
1½ cups (375 ml) soy milk, plus extra if needed
2 teaspoons ground cinnamon
2 teaspoons baking powder
Small amount of olive oil, for cooking
Chopped fruit, to serve
100% natural nut butter of your choice, at room temperature or melted slightly, to serve

1. Combine the oats, banana, soy milk, cinnamon and baking powder in a blender. Blend for 1 minute or until smooth.
2. Set aside for 5 minutes to rest and thicken. If the batter is too thick for your liking, stir in some extra soy milk until the batter reaches your desired consistency.
3. Heat a small amount of oil in a medium frying pan over medium heat. Pour in the pancake batter until it fills three-quarters of the pan. Cook for 2 minutes, until you start to see bubbles forming on the surface. Flip the pancake and cook for another 2–4 minutes, until golden.

4. Remove the pancake from the pan and continue until all the batter is used. If you have a large frying pan or griddle pan you could cook more than one at a time.

5. Serve the pancakes warm, topped with chopped fruit and drizzled with nut butter.

CHICKPEA SCRAMBLE (with video)

This is a hearty vegan breakfast dish. Try swapping out your usual scrambled eggs and have a go at a chickpea scramble instead. You can also experiment by adding different herbs and spices.

Serves 4

Prep Time: 10 minutes
Cooking Time: 10 minutes

2 × 400 g tins chickpeas, rinsed and drained
½ cup (125 ml) soy milk
2 teaspoons ground turmeric
1 teaspoon ground cumin
1 teaspoon olive oil
4 thick slices sourdough bread
1 avocado
Fresh herbs and dried chilli flakes, to serve (optional)

1. Place the chickpeas into a mixing bowl and use a fork to roughly mash. Add half the soy milk and mash into the chickpeas, then add the remaining soy milk and continue mashing to combine. Stir in the turmeric and cumin, and season with salt and pepper if desired.
2. Heat the oil in a non-stick frying pan over medium heat. Add the mashed chickpea mixture and cook for about 10 minutes, stirring occasionally, until the mixture starts to dry out and has a slightly crispy texture.
3. Meanwhile, toast the bread. Cool slightly, then mash the avocado onto the toast. Top with the scrambled chickpea mixture. Sprinkle with fresh herbs and chilli flakes to serve, if desired.

CHOC CHIA PUDDING

This chia pudding will satisfy any chocolate craving, so even though it is a healthy breakfast, it would make a delicious treat any time. You could serve it with other toppings that pair well with chocolate, such as raspberries, strawberries, 100 per cent natural almond butter or a sprinkle of crunchy granola. The cocoa powder adds a rich bitter chocolate taste, which is offset by the sweet banana. If you don't want to use banana, you may want to add a tiny drizzle of honey or naturally sweetened yoghurt.

Serves 4

Prep Time: 5 minutes + overnight refrigeration

½ cup (100 g) chia seeds
2½ cups (625 ml) milk
1 tablespoon cocoa powder
2 bananas, sliced, to serve

1. Place the chia seeds, milk and cocoa into a bowl. Stir well to combine, then cover and refrigerate overnight.
2. In the morning, give the chia pudding a good stir. Divide between 4 serving bowls or glasses.
3. Top with the banana (or topping of your choice) and serve.

CHIA PUDDING PARFAIT
Try this parfait as a variation.

Place ½ cup (100 g) chia seeds and 2 cups (500 ml) milk in a bowl. Stir well to combine, cover and refrigerate overnight. To serve, give the mixture a good stir, then layer into 4 glasses, with 2 cups (560 g) plain Greek yoghurt divided between the layers. Top with sliced strawberries to serve.

CORN FRITTERS

Corn fritters are very versatile – serve them for breakfast, lunch, dinner or for a snack. They can be prepared in advance and packed into school or work lunchboxes, or whipped up for an after school snack. Add some chopped red chilli or dried chilli flakes for an extra kick, or serve with your favourite chutney.

Makes 16–20

Prep Time: 10 minutes
Cooking Time: 15 minutes

2 corn cobs, husks and silk removed
2 eggs
½ cup (125 ml) milk
1 small red capsicum, finely chopped
Handful of fresh coriander leaves and stalks, chopped
1 cup (160 g) wholemeal self-raising flour
3 tablespoons olive oil

1. Use a small sharp knife to cut the kernels from the corn cobs.
2. Place the eggs and milk into a large bowl and whisk to combine. Stir in the corn kernels, capsicum and coriander. Add the flour and stir gently until just combined.
3. Heat 1 tablespoon of olive oil in a large frying pan over medium-high heat. Using about 2 tablespoons of batter for each fritter, drop a few piles into the pan and flatten slightly. Cook for 2–3 minutes each side, until golden brown. Transfer to a plate.
4. Heat another tablespoon of olive oil in the frying pan. Continue to cook the fritters in batches until all of the batter has been used up, adding more oil for the last batch as needed. Serve warm.

PANCAKE TRAY BAKE (with video)

If you are making breakfast for a crowd, why not give this pancake tray bake a try? You can place this into the oven and in 20 minutes breakfast will be ready – rather than standing over a hot stove and flipping pancakes. Top with any fruit of your choice.

Serves 6

Prep Time: 10 minutes
Cooking Time: 20 minutes

1⅓ cups (330 ml) milk
1½ tablespoons olive oil
1 egg
2 tablespoons honey
1¼ cups (200 g) wholemeal self-raising flour
1 teaspoon baking powder
1 teaspoon ground cinnamon
Seasonal fruit, thinly sliced, plus extra to serve
Greek yoghurt, to serve

1. Preheat the oven to 180°C (fan-forced).
2. Place the milk, olive oil, egg and honey into a large jug. Whisk well to combine.
3. Combine the flour, baking powder and cinnamon in a large mixing bowl. Make a well in the centre of the flour mixture. Pour the wet ingredients into the dry ingredients. Stir well to combine and ensure no lumps remain.
4. Pour the pancake batter mixture into a large baking dish (approx. 30 cm × 20 cm), lined with baking paper and/or greased with olive oil. Top the pancake batter with sliced fruit. Bake for 20 minutes until golden and fluffy.
5. Cut the pancake into 6 portions and arrange onto serving plates. Serve topped with extra sliced fruit and a generous dollop of Greek yoghurt.

BLUEBERRY PANCAKES

These pancakes can be whipped up in no time by using a blender or a food processor. Alternatively, they can also be made the old-fashioned way by combining the wet ingredients together and then adding to the dry ingredients. Serve with whatever fruit is in season!

Serves 4

Prep Time: 5 minutes
Cooking Time: 20 minutes

1½ cups (180 g) ground almonds
½ cup (80 g) wholemeal plain flour
1 teaspoon baking powder
4 eggs
2 overripe bananas
½ cup (125 ml) skim milk
1 cup (150 g) blueberries (fresh, or thawed if using frozen)
Olive oil spray
Greek yoghurt, to serve
Mixed fruit, chopped, to serve

1. Combine the ground almonds, flour, baking powder, eggs, bananas and milk in a blender or food processor. Blend until well combined, without any lumps. Transfer the mixture to a jug and stir through the blueberries.
2. Spray a medium frying pan with olive oil spray then heat over medium heat. Pour batter from the jug into the pan to make small pancakes, about 5–6 cm in diameter. Cook for about 2 minutes, until you see bubbles start to form on the surface. Flip the pancakes and cook for another 2–3 minutes, until golden.
3. Continue cooking the pancakes in batches until all the batter is used.
4. Serve the pancakes warm, topped with Greek yoghurt and fruit.

ON-THE-GO STRAWBERRY BREAKFAST PARFAIT (with video)

A fancier way to prepare your overnight oats! This recipe uses strawberries, but you could swap for any fruit or berry that is in season when you choose to try this recipe. The peanut butter can also be swapped for any other nut butter that you prefer. Don't worry if the layers in your jar aren't perfect – it will still taste delicious!

Serves 4

Prep Time: 10 minutes + 4 hours soaking, or overnight refrigeration

2 cups (180 g) rolled oats
1½ cups (375 ml) milk
12 strawberries
⅓ cup (45 g) hulled hemp seeds
2 cups (560 g) Greek yoghurt
100% natural peanut butter, to serve

1. Place the rolled oats and milk into a bowl and stir to combine. Place into the fridge for at least 4 hours (or up to 8) to allow the oats to soak up the liquid.
2. When it is time to assemble, cut the strawberries into thin slices. Grab 4 clean glass jars with lids.
3. Divide half the overnight oats between the jars. Sprinkle 1 tablespoon of hemp seeds into each jar.
   Divide half the strawberries between each jar, then half the yoghurt. Spoon the remaining oats into the jars.
4. Top each with a spoonful of peanut butter, and the remaining Greek yoghurt and strawberries. Screw on the lids, and the breakfast is ready to grab and go.

Note: If taking with you (i.e. to work), transport in a chiller bag and refrigerate until time to eat.

BREAKFAST BAGELS

A fun breakfast idea, perfect to make with the whole family on the weekend.

Serves 4

Prep Time: 5 minutes
Cooking Time: 10 minutes

4 wholegrain seeded bagels, halved horizontally
1 tablespoon olive oil
4 eggs
1 avocado, mashed
250 g cherry tomatoes, halved
¼ red onion, thinly sliced

1. Lightly toast the bagel halves, either in a toaster or under the grill.
2. Meanwhile, heat the olive oil in a large frying pan over medium heat. Crack in the eggs and fry for 1–2 minutes. Reduce the heat to low and place a lid over the pan. Continue to cook the eggs sunny side up for another 3–4 minutes, until cooked to your liking.
3. Spread the bagel halves evenly with avocado. Place the bottom half of each of the bagels onto four serving plates. Top with the cherry tomatoes and red onion.
4. To serve, place an egg onto each bagel, then put the bagel lids on top.

CARROT CAKE OVERNIGHT OATS

Here we have all the yummy flavours of carrot cake transformed into a bowl of oats. It is a comforting and satisfying breakfast that can be prepared quickly the night before. These flavours would also work well mixed into a bowl of warm cooked porridge.

Serves 4

Prep Time: 10 minutes + overnight refrigeration

2 cups (180 g) rolled oats
2 teaspoons chia seeds
2 cups (500 ml) skim milk
½ cup (140 g) Greek yoghurt, plus extra to serve
2 carrots, grated
2 teaspoons ground cinnamon
½ teaspoon ground nutmeg
Sprinkle of pepitas

1. Place the oats, chia seeds, milk, yoghurt, grated carrot, cinnamon and nutmeg into a bowl. Stir well to combine, then cover and refrigerate overnight to soak.
2. To serve, divide the carrot cake oats between serving bowls and top with a dollop of Greek yoghurt and a sprinkle of pepitas.

EASY GRANOLA (with video)

A fast and easy recipe that results in a delicious batch of homemade granola – perfect for quick weekday breakfasts! Much healthier than the store-bought versions that can be full of sugar. Feel free to substitute any nuts and seeds that you have in the pantry. You can also use this granola to make the 'Easy Breakfast Cookies' recipe on page 170.

Serves 8 (makes 1 large jar)

Prep Time: 10 minutes
Cooking Time: 30 minutes

1½ cups (135 g) rolled oats
½ cup (75 g) raw cashews
½ cup (80 g) raw almonds
1 tablespoon shredded coconut
½ cup (75 g) mixed seeds (such as pepitas and sunflower seeds)
¼ cup (60 ml) olive oil
1 tablespoon honey
Sprinkle of ground cinnamon

1. Preheat the oven to 190°C (fan-forced). Line a large rimmed baking tray with baking paper
2. Place the oats, cashews, almonds, coconut and seeds into a large mixing bowl.
3. Combine the olive oil and honey in a small bowl. Heat in the microwave for 10–20 seconds, until the honey is runny. Stir to combine, then pour over the dry ingredients. Stir well to ensure everything is combined and coated.

4. Transfer the granola to the prepared tray and spread it out evenly. Bake for 15 minutes, then remove from the oven and gently stir with a spoon. This will help it to cook evenly. Bake for a further 10–15 minutes, until golden brown.

5. Remove from the oven and sprinkle with cinnamon. Allow to cool completely, then transfer to an airtight jar. Keep for up to 1 month in the pantry.

EASY BREAKFAST COOKIES (with video)

This recipe has minimal ingredients, is quick and simple to make, and results in a yummy cookie that is perfect to pack as part of an on-the-go breakfast or as a lunchbox snack – what more could you ask for? You could get creative with this recipe and add some chopped dried fruit, replace the nuts with some nut butter for flavour, or even sprinkle pepitas, sunflower or chia seeds over the top before baking.

Makes 12

Prep Time: 10 minutes
Cooking Time: 20 minutes

2 ripe bananas
1½ cups (135 g) sugar-free muesli or rolled oats (or Easy Granola – page 168)
¼ cup (25 g) walnuts, roasted, coarsely chopped

1. Preheat the oven to 180°C (fan-forced). Line 2 baking trays with baking paper.
2. Place the bananas into a mixing bowl and mash with a fork until smooth. Add the muesli and walnuts and stir well to combine.
3. Scoop tablespoons of mixture onto the trays. Use the back of a spoon to flatten into a cookie shape.
4. Bake for 15–20 minutes, until lightly golden. Cool on the trays for 5 minutes, then transfer to a wire rack to cool completely. Store in an airtight container for up to 3 days.

BAKED OATS

Oats are such a healthy and versatile breakfast ingredient. Baked oats have a consistency similar to a warm cake or pudding. This is a versatile recipe as you can top them with any ingredients that you fancy. If preparing in advance, you can store the batter in the fridge for 1–2 days and then bake just before eating. Alternatively you can bake these ahead of time and enjoy cold, or reheat just before serving.

Serves 4

Prep Time: 5 minutes
Cooking Time: 20 minutes

2 cups (180 g) rolled oats
2 small bananas
2 eggs
2 teaspoons baking powder
½ cup (125 ml) milk
Toppings of your choice, to serve (see Note)

1. Preheat the oven to 180°C (fan-forced).
2. Place the oats into a blender and use the pulse button to blend in short bursts, until the oats resemble a rough flour consistency.
3. Add the bananas, eggs, baking powder and milk. Blend for 1–2 minutes, until smooth.
4. Pour the mixture into 4 small ramekins or ovenproof dishes (or a small baking dish). Stand the ramekins on a baking tray.
5. Bake for 15–20 minutes, until the mixture has risen and is slightly firm to the touch. Depending on the size and shape of your dish, you may prefer to cook slightly longer. If you prefer a fudgy texture you can cook for slightly less time.
6. Set aside to cool slightly, then serve with your chosen toppings.

Note: You can top with sliced banana, berries, yoghurt, honey, nut butter or hemp seeds.

ONE-PAN FAST FRITTATA

This is a simple frittata recipe that you can whip up quickly without having to turn on your oven. Perfect for a weekend breakfast, and substantial enough to have as a light meal for lunch or dinner. It works well with the small beans and peas, but you could always swap for your preferred choice of vegetable, just make sure you slice it nice and small and pre-cook slightly.

Serves 4

Prep Time: 10 minutes
Cooking Time: 12 minutes

300 g shelled frozen edamame
200 g frozen baby peas
8 eggs
Large handful of flat-leaf parsley leaves, torn
2 tablespoons olive oil
4 spring onions, sliced
Crumbled feta, to serve
Toasted grainy bread, to serve (gluten-free if necessary)

1. Place the frozen edamame and peas in a bowl and cover with boiling water. Stand for a couple of minutes, until thawed. Drain well.
2. Crack the eggs into a large jug and whisk well. Add the edamame, peas and parsley.
3. Heat the olive oil in a non-stick frying pan over medium heat. Add the spring onions and fry for a couple of minutes, until softened. Pour the egg mixture into the pan. Swirl the pan carefully to distribute the ingredients evenly.
4. Cook, covered, for about 10 minutes. When ready, the bottom of the frittata should be set and lightly golden (you can use a spatula to lift up the side and look underneath) and the middle of the frittata should be puffed up and no longer wobbly.
5. To serve, slide the frittata gently out of the pan and onto a plate. Scatter over some feta and season with freshly ground black pepper if desired. Serve immediately with toast.

SHAKSHUKA

This dish is on breakfast menus all over Israel, and it's easy to fall in love with it for its tasty and healthy properties. It's also hearty enough to have for lunch or dinner and is a ripper for serving to friends or family.

Serves 4

Prep Time: 10 minutes
Cooking Time: 15 minutes

1 teaspoon olive oil
4 cloves garlic, crushed
½ brown onion, diced
2 teaspoons chopped fresh chilli (or dried chilli flakes)
3 teaspoons paprika
3 teaspoons ground cumin
2 × 400 g tins crushed tomatoes
1 red capsicum, chopped
4 eggs
1 large handful of basil leaves, baby rocket or baby spinach
Toasted grainy bread, to serve (gluten-free if necessary)

1. Heat the oil in a large frying pan over medium heat. Add the garlic, onion, chilli and spices and cook for 2 minutes, until aromatic.
2. Add the tomato and capsicum and cook for 5 minutes, until soft.
3. Create four wells in the tomato mixture, then crack an egg into each well. Cover the pan with a lid and cook for 5–7 minutes, until the egg whites are firm with a runny yolk (or to your liking).
4. Top with basil, rocket or baby spinach and serve with toast.

Note: You could replace the tinned tomatoes with about 3 cups roughly chopped fresh tomatoes. It's a great way to use up tomatoes that are overripe and extra juicy.

PUMPKIN AND RICOTTA FRITTATA

Frittata can be made in advance and stored in the fridge for a quick breakfast (or even lunch or dinner!). You can substitute whatever vegetables you have in your fridge, but the flavour combination of the ingredients in this version is delicious! Use firm ricotta from the deli counter, not smooth ricotta from a tub.

Serves 6–8

Prep Time: 15 minutes
Cooking Time: 50 minutes

¼ butternut pumpkin (about 400 g), peeled, seeded, cut into
    small cubes
7 eggs
¾ cup (180 ml) milk
1¼ cups (250 g) fresh ricotta (from the deli counter)
1 zucchini, chopped
5 sun-dried tomato halves, sliced into thin strips
Handful of flat-leaf parsley leaves, plus extra to serve

1. Preheat the oven to 200°C (fan-forced). Line a baking tray with baking paper. Lightly grease a 20 cm square non-stick cake tin.
2. Place the pumpkin onto a baking tray, and roast for 10 minutes. Meanwhile, place the eggs and milk into a mixing bowl. Whisk well to combine.
3. Remove the pumpkin from the oven and set aside to cool for a few minutes.
4. Reserve a small amount of the ricotta for topping, then break the rest into large chunks. Stir into the egg mixture, then stir in the pumpkin, zucchini and sun-dried tomatoes.
5. Pour the egg mixture into the prepared tin. Sprinkle with parsley, then dot the reserved ricotta over the top.
6. Bake for 30–40 minutes, until puffed up, set and lightly golden on top. Sprinkle with extra parsley and cut into pieces to serve.

SOUPS, SALADS AND SIDES

BUTTERNUT PUMPKIN SOUP

Using butternut pumpkin for this recipe creates a sweet and creamy soup. It's a perfect dish for the cooler months. Soup is also great to make in a large batch and store in the fridge or freezer for pre-made meals throughout the week. Serve with crispy toasted wholegrain bread.

Serves 6

Prep Time: 15 minutes
Cooking Time: 25 minutes

1 tablespoon olive oil
1 clove garlic, crushed
1 brown onion, chopped
½ large butternut pumpkin (about 1 kg), peeled, seeded and chopped
3 small slices fresh turmeric (skin on), or 1 teaspoon ground turmeric
1 teaspoon ground cumin
4 cups (1 litre) vegetable stock
Greek yoghurt, to serve (optional)

1. Heat the olive oil in a large saucepan over medium heat. Add the garlic and onion and cook for 5 minutes, stirring occasionally, until soft.
2. Add the pumpkin, turmeric and cumin. Stir to combine and cook for a couple of minutes. Pour over the vegetable stock and turn up the heat to bring to the boil.
3. Reduce the heat and simmer the soup for 15 minutes or until the pumpkin is tender and falling apart when stirred.
4. Remove the soup from the heat and use a stick blender to blend the soup until smooth. Alternatively, allow the soup to cool slightly before blending in batches in a blender.
5. Return the soup to the pan to heat through if necessary. Divide between serving bowls and top with a dollop of Greek yoghurt, if using, and some freshly ground black pepper if desired.

SLOW COOKER MINESTRONE

Minestrone is a great winter staple, and it's even better when it takes very little effort to prepare it in a slow cooker. Feel free to add in whatever vegetables and beans you already have at home. If you have the rind of a piece of parmesan left in your fridge, you can add it to this soup to give it a delicious rich flavour.

Serves 6

Prep Time: 15 minutes
Cooking Time: 3½ or 6½ hours

1 tablespoon olive oil
1 red onion, finely chopped
1 clove garlic, crushed
1 large carrot, chopped
2 sticks celery, chopped
1 bulb fennel, chopped
400 g tin crushed tomatoes
400 g tin cannellini beans, rinsed and drained
4 cups (1 litre) vegetable stock
1 bunch basil, leaves picked
1 piece parmesan rind (optional)
1 cup (180 g) wholemeal pasta
1 bunch kale, stems removed, leaves chopped

1. Turn the slow cooker on to the high setting. Combine the olive oil and onion in the slow cooker so it starts cooking while you chop up the remaining ingredients. Add the garlic.
2. Add the carrot, celery, fennel, tomatoes, cannellini beans, stock, 6 cups (1.5 litres) water, basil leaves and parmesan rind, if using. Stir to combine.
3. Cover and cook for 3 hours on high (or 6 hours on low if you prefer).

4. If the soup has been cooking on low, turn the setting to high. Add the pasta, cover and cook for 15–20 minutes, until al dente (slightly firm to the bite). The pasta will take 15–20 minutes if it is a small shape such as small macaroni, or about 30 minutes if it is a larger shape such as penne or rigatoni.

5. Stir through the kale leaves to wilt, and turn off the slow cooker. Remove the parmesan rind. Divide the soup between serving bowls and serve seasoned with freshly ground black pepper if desired.

TOMATO SOUP

A delicious, comforting and warming winter soup that is surprisingly easy to make. The addition of the potato makes this soup nice and creamy. Roasting adds a depth of flavour to the tomatoes which may not be optimum in winter.

Serves 4

Prep Time: 10 minutes
Cooking Time: 40 minutes

1 kg ripe Roma tomatoes, halved
3 tablespoons olive oil
1 brown onion, chopped
2 cloves garlic, crushed
2 potatoes, chopped
¼ cup (70 g) tomato paste
2 cups (500 ml) vegetable stock

1. Preheat the oven to 200°C (fan-forced). Line a baking tray with baking paper.
2. Place the tomatoes onto the prepared tray and drizzle with 1 tablespoon of the oil. Bake for 20–25 minutes, until softened and lightly browned.
3. Meanwhile, heat the remaining oil in a large saucepan over medium-high heat. Add the onion and garlic and cook for 2–3 minutes, until just soft. Add the potato and cook, stirring occasionally, for 10 minutes. Stir in the tomato paste, stock and 1 cup (250 ml) water. Bring to the boil.
4. Cover the saucepan with a lid and reduce the heat to low. Simmer for 15 minutes or until the potatoes are soft.
5. Add the roasted tomatoes to the soup. Remove the soup from the heat and use a stick blender to blend until smooth. Alternatively, allow the soup to cool slightly before blending in batches in a blender. Reheat gently if necessary, and serve.

CORN CHOWDER (with video)

This hearty and delicious winter soup is quick and easy to prepare for a warming weeknight dinner! If you would like to make a vegan version of this dish you can swap the milk for a plant-based version such as soy milk.

Serves 4

Prep Time: 10 minutes
Cooking Time: 30 minutes

2 tablespoons olive oil
1 brown onion, chopped
2 cloves garlic, crushed
1 large red capsicum, chopped
1 kg frozen corn kernels
Sprinkle of paprika, to taste
2 cups (500 ml) milk
400 g tin red kidney beans, rinsed and drained
Handful of coriander leaves, plus extra to serve

1. Heat the oil in a large saucepan over medium heat. Add the onion and garlic and cook for 5 minutes, stirring occasionally, until soft. Stir in the capsicum and cook for another couple of minutes.
2. Turn the heat up to medium-high and stir in the frozen corn. Season with paprika, salt and freshly ground black pepper if desired.
3. Add the milk and bring just to a simmer, then reduce the heat to medium-low and cook for 15 minutes, stirring every 5 minutes.
4. Transfer about one-third of the soup to a blender. Cool slightly, then blend until smooth. (Alternatively, place one-third of the soup into a bowl and use a stick blender for this step.)
5. Return the blended soup to the saucepan and stir to combine. Add the red kidney beans and the coriander. Stir through the soup, then heat through over medium heat for 5 minutes.
6. Ladle into serving bowls and top with extra coriander to serve.

NEXT LEVEL GREEK SALAD

Level up the everyday Greek salad with this fresh and flavoursome recipe. The feta is grilled, which adds a lovely flavour, and the beans and chickpeas add a hit of protein. The quick pickled onions add even more flavour and texture. You could substitute the feta with some grilled haloumi drizzled with honey, if you like.

Serves 6

Prep Time: 15 minutes
Cooking Time: 5 minutes

200 g block Greek feta, cut into six pieces
2 tablespoons olive oil
1 bunch flat-leaf parsley, leaves chopped
1 red capsicum, chopped
1 large tomato, chopped
400 g tin chickpeas, rinsed and drained
400 g tin red kidney beans, rinsed and drained
1 Lebanese cucumber, chopped
2 tablespoons pitted black olives
2 tablespoons Quick Pickled Onions (see page 201)
Sprinkle of dried oregano
Finely grated zest and juice of 1 lemon

1. Heat a small char-grill pan over medium heat. Brush the feta with 1 tablespoon of the olive oil and cook for 1 minute on each side, until golden.
2. Meanwhile combine the remaining oil and all the other ingredients in a large salad bowl. Toss gently to combine.
3. Serve the char-grilled feta immediately, accompanied by the Greek salad.

MAPLE ROAST PUMPKIN SALAD

A simple yet delicious side dish to serve alongside your chosen protein source. This salad can be enjoyed warm once the pumpkin is taken out of the oven, or it is just as yummy cold out of the fridge the next day.

Serves 4–6

Prep Time: 10 minutes
Cooking Time: 35 minutes

¼ large Kent pumpkin (about 1 kg), seeded, sliced into large pieces
¼ cup (60 ml) olive oil
1 tablespoon pure maple syrup (not maple-flavoured syrup)
1 tablespoon smoked paprika
60 g bag baby rocket
½ red onion, thinly sliced
200 g Greek feta

1. Preheat the oven to 200°C (fan-forced). Line 2 baking trays with baking paper.
2. Place the pumpkin slices onto the baking trays. Drizzle with the olive oil and maple syrup, then use your hands to combine and coat both sides of the pumpkin.
3. Spread out and arrange in a single layer. Sprinkle with paprika and season with salt and freshly ground black pepper if desired.
4. Roast for 25–35 minutes, until the pumpkin is soft and the edges are golden brown. Cool slightly.
5. Arrange the rocket and red onion in a salad bowl. Top with the maple roast pumpkin. Crumble the feta over the top and serve.

HERBY COUSCOUS SALAD

This recipe takes simple ingredients and turns them into a flavoursome and exciting salad, one that you could proudly take along to a summer get-together or picnic! Enjoy this alongside a serve of lean protein of your choice. This salad also packs well for lunch.

Serves 4

Prep Time: 15 minutes
Cooking Time: 5 minutes

2 cups (400 g) wholemeal couscous
2⅔ cups (660 ml) boiling water
2 tablespoons olive oil
3 large zucchini, cut into thick slices
2 cups mixed lettuce leaves
Handful of fresh herbs
¼ cup (35 g) shelled pistachios, toasted
¼ cup (40 g) pine nuts, toasted
Dried chilli flakes, to serve (optional)

Herby dressing
2 cups fresh herbs (such as parsley and mint, but use what you have)
2 cloves garlic
⅓ cup (80 ml) olive oil

1. Place the couscous into a large bowl and pour over the boiling water. Cover tightly and stand for 5–10 minutes, until all the water has been absorbed. Fluff the couscous with a fork to separate the grains, then set aside.
2. To make the Herby dressing: Place the ingredients into a blender and blend until smooth. Add a little warm water if necessary, to combine the ingredients into a smooth runny mixture. Season with freshly ground black pepper to taste.
3. Pour the Herby dressing over the couscous and use a fork to mix well.

4. Heat the olive oil in a large non-stick frying pan. Add the zucchini and cook for 1–2 minutes each side, until golden.

5. Place the lettuce leaves into a large salad bowl. Top with the herby couscous, and arrange the zucchini slices over the couscous. Scatter the herbs over, then sprinkle with the toasted pistachios and pine nuts. Sprinkle with chilli flakes, if using, and serve.

SUMMER PASTA SALAD (with video)

All the colours of Christmas combined in one delicious pasta salad!
This salad not only looks good but tastes great too! This salad is
perfect to pack on a picnic, or to take with you to a holiday gathering.
Serve this as a side salad with your choice of lean protein.

Serves 6

Prep Time: 10 minutes
Cooking Time: 15 minutes

400 g wholemeal spiral pasta
2 tablespoons Homemade Basil Pesto (see page 200)
500 g cherry or 400 g grape tomatoes, quartered
200 g cherry bocconcini, halved
1 bunch basil, leaves picked

1. Bring a large saucepan of water to the boil over high heat. Add the
   pasta and cook for about 12 minutes, or until al dente (still slightly
   firm to the bite).
2. When the pasta is cooked, reserve ½ cup (125 ml) of the pasta
   water, then drain. Return the pasta to the large saucepan or a
   large salad bowl.
3. Add the pesto to the pasta, as well as some of the pasta water.
   Stir well to ensure the pasta is evenly coated, adding more of the
   reserved pasta water if necessary. Add the tomatoes, bocconcini
   and basil leaves. Stir gently to combine.
4. Serve pasta salad immediately while it is warm, or store in the fridge
   until ready to serve cold.

SUMMER NECTARINE SALAD

A bright and colourful summer salad – perfect to make on a hot summer evening. If you have the barbecue going you can grill the nectarine and haloumi on the barbecue, but a char-grill pan works just as well. You can substitute the vegetables in this salad for any that you already have on hand in your fridge. The creamy dressing adds lots of delicious flavour!

Serves 4

Prep Time: 15 minutes
Cooking Time: 10 minutes

1 large bag (120 g) mixed salad leaves
½ red onion, thinly sliced
1 large red capsicum, thinly sliced
250 g cherry tomatoes, halved
1 Lebanese cucumber, chopped
400 g tin butter beans, rinsed and drained
1 avocado, chopped
2 large handfuls of flat-leaf parsley leaves, chopped
4 yellow nectarines, cut into wedges
200 g haloumi, cut into thick slices

Dressing
⅓ cup (80 ml) olive oil
2 tablespoons tahini
Juice of 1 large lemon
2 cloves garlic, crushed
1 teaspoon wholegrain mustard
2 tablespoons honey

1. To make the dressing, combine all the dressing ingredients in a small jar. Screw the lid on tight and shake well to combine.
2. Arrange the salad leaves in a large salad bowl and top with the onion, capsicum, cherry tomatoes, cucumber, butter beans, avocado and parsley.
3. Heat a char-grill pan (or barbecue) over medium-high heat. Add the nectarine and haloumi and cook for 2–3 minutes on each side until lightly charred and caramelised. Arrange on top of the salad.
4. Drizzle with the dressing and serve immediately.

CREAMY CHICKPEA COLESLAW

A simple salad that can be eaten as a substantial lunch on its own or served as a side salad with some grilled fish or meat. Why not make up a big bowl to take to your next summer barbecue gathering and impress your friends?

Serves 4 (or 6 as a side salad)

Prep Time: 10 minutes

1 bag dry coleslaw mix (approx. 400 g)
1 spring onion, chopped
400 g tin of chickpeas, drained and rinsed

Creamy dressing
2 tablespoons tahini
1 tablespoon Dijon mustard
¼ cup (60 ml) lemon juice

1. Place the coleslaw mix, spring onion and chickpeas in a large bowl.
2. To make the creamy dressing, combine the tahini, mustard and lemon juice in a small bowl. Whisk with a fork until well combined. Add one tablespoon of warm water to help bring the ingredients together and to thin out the dressing. Season with freshly ground black pepper, if desired.
3. Pour the dressing over the coleslaw ingredients. Toss to combine well and coat evenly with the dressing.

FRESH VERMICELLI NOODLE SALAD

This salad is made with raw vegetables which makes it quick and easy.
It is delicious for lunch or dinner on hot days.

Serves 4

Prep Time: 15 minutes
Cooking Time: 5 minutes

250 g rice vermicelli noodles
1 teaspoon olive oil
400 g firm tofu, sliced into thin strips
1 zucchini
1 carrot
1 red capsicum, sliced thinly
2 sticks celery, sliced thinly
Handful of chives, chopped
Handful of coriander leaves, chopped
Handful of mint leaves, chopped
Small handful of unsalted roasted cashews, chopped

Dressing
2 tablespoons 100% natural peanut butter
Juice of 1 lime
1 tablespoon gluten-free soy sauce (or tamari)
1 teaspoon sriracha
1 teaspoon finely grated ginger

1. Place the noodles into a large bowl. Cover with boiling water and
   stand for 5 minutes, until softened. Drain into a colander and rinse
   under cold running water. Drain well and set aside.
2. Heat the olive oil in a non-stick frying pan over medium heat. Add
   the tofu strips and fry for 5 minutes, turning regularly, until golden.
   Set aside.

3. Meanwhile, use a vegetable peeler to create long thin ribbons of the zucchini and carrot. Place into a large salad bowl with the capsicum, celery, chives, coriander and mint. Add the noodles and tofu.
4. To make the dressing, combine all the dressing ingredients in a small bowl and stir to combine. Add up to ¼ cup (60 ml) warm water, a little at a time, to help the dressing come together.
5. Pour the dressing over the salad. Use tongs to toss and combine all the ingredients together. Sprinkle the cashews over the top and serve.

Note: You could also use a julienne peeler or vegetable spiraliser to create thin veggie strips.

ROAST CARROT SALAD

A perfect dish to make in a large quantity and add to lunches and meals throughout the week. Delicious eaten either hot or cold! If you would like a vegan option, simply omit the honey or replace with sweetener of your choice.

Serves 4

Prep Time: 15 minutes
Cooking Time: 25 minutes

6 carrots, skin on, cut into finger-sized pieces
1 teaspoon olive oil
1 teaspoon ground sumac
¼ cup (25 g) walnuts, chopped
Handful of flat-leaf parsley leaves
Seeds of 1 pomegranate

Dressing
1 teaspoon honey
Finely grated zest and juice of 1 lemon
1 tablespoon red wine vinegar
1 teaspoon olive oil

1. Preheat the oven to 180°C (fan-forced). Place the carrots onto a large baking tray and sprinkle with olive oil and sumac. Turn to coat then spread out in an even layer.
2. Roast for 15 minutes. Add the walnuts to the tray and roast for another 5–10 minutes, until golden.
3. To make the dressing, place the ingredients into a small jar. Screw the lid on tight and shake well to combine.
4. Transfer the roasted carrots and walnuts to a serving dish. Add the parsley and pomegranate seeds to the carrots, then pour over the dressing. Toss to combine, then serve.

MEDITERRANEAN PASTA SALAD (with video)

This is a flavoursome pasta salad, perfect served as a side to a serve of lean protein. Alternatively, you could add a couple of tins of chickpeas and pack this for a hearty weekday lunch. It works well served as a warm salad, or cold from the fridge.

Serves 6–8 as a side

Prep Time: 15 minutes
Cooking Time: 40 minutes

1–2 zucchini, chopped
1 red capsicum, chopped
1 large eggplant, chopped
10 button mushrooms, halved
1 red onion, chopped
1 tablespoon olive oil
2 cloves garlic, crushed
500 g wholemeal spiral pasta
100 g feta, chopped into small pieces
1 bunch basil, leaves picked

Dressing
¼ cup (60 ml) olive oil
Juice of 1 lemon
Sprinkle each of dried parsley, thyme and oregano
Sprinkle of dried chilli flakes

1. Preheat the oven to 200°C (fan-forced). Line 2 large baking trays with baking paper.
2. Toss the vegetables with the oil and garlic to coat. Spread onto the baking trays. Roast for 25 minutes, turning the vegetables halfway through cooking, until tender and lightly browned. Set aside to cool slightly.
3. Meanwhile, to make the dressing, combine the ingredients in a jar and season lightly with salt and pepper if desired. Tighten the lid then shake well to combine.

4. Transfer the roasted vegetables into a large salad bowl. Pour in half of the dressing and toss to combine. Cover and set aside for the vegetables to soak up the dressing while the pasta cooks.

5. Meanwhile, bring a large saucepan of water to the boil over high heat. Add the pasta and cook for about 12 minutes, until al dente (still slightly firm to the bite). Drain the pasta into a colander and rinse lightly under warm running water. Drain well.

6. Transfer the pasta to the bowl with the roasted vegetables. Pour in the remaining dressing, feta and basil leaves. Mix the pasta salad well to combine and ensure everything is coated in the dressing. Serve warm, or refrigerate until required.

Note: Keep in mind that the capsicum and mushrooms will cook quickly, so cut these into larger chunks. The zucchini, eggplant and onion will take a bit longer to cook, so cut these into slightly smaller chunks.

CHRISTMAS RICE PILAF (with video)

This dish is easier to prepare than it looks! Impress friends and family when you serve this dish at a get-together over the festive season! The finished dish looks beautiful with the sprinkle of red jewel-like pomegranate seeds and the green herb leaves. It is perfect as a side dish to a lean serve of protein.

Serves 6 as a side

Prep Time: 15 minutes
Cooking Time: 30 minutes + 10 minutes standing

2 tablespoons olive oil
2 cloves garlic, crushed
1 brown onion, chopped
¼ teaspoon ground cinnamon
¼ teaspoon ground cardamom
¼ teaspoon ground cumin
1 cup (200 g) jasmine rice
1¾ cups (430 ml) vegetable stock
½ cup (75 g) dried apricots, chopped
Large handful of flat-leaf parsley leaves, chopped
Large handful of coriander leaves, chopped
Seeds of 1 pomegranate
½ cup (70 g) slivered almonds, toasted

1. Heat the oil in a large saucepan over medium-high heat. Add the garlic and onion and cook for 5 minutes, until the onion is soft.
2. Stir in the cinnamon, cardamom, cumin and rice. Season with freshly ground black pepper if desired. Cook for another 5 minutes to toast the rice, stirring occasionally. Pour in the vegetable stock and stir to combine. Cover with a lid and bring to a simmer.

3. Add the dried apricots, then cover the pan with the lid again. Reduce the heat to medium-low and cook for 15 minutes, until the rice has absorbed the liquid. Leave the lid on during this time to ensure the liquid doesn't evaporate.

4. Turn off the heat and stand, covered, for 10 minutes. Use a fork to fluff up the rice. Top the rice pilaf with the parsley and coriander, pomegranate seeds and slivered almonds. Serve immediately.

ONE-PAN ROASTED EGGPLANT (with video)

A simple yet delicious one-pan dish, perfect to whip up while eggplants are in season. Serve this alongside a grilled lean protein source, a rocket salad, and some wholemeal couscous or quinoa. Leftovers will store well in the fridge for up to one week and make for a great packed lunch.

Serves 4

Prep Time: 10 minutes
Cooking Time: 55 minutes

2 large eggplants, halved lengthways
3 tablespoons olive oil
2 cloves garlic, crushed
1 brown onion, chopped
1 tablespoon balsamic vinegar
1 heaped tablespoon tomato paste
50 g (1 small box) sultanas
250 g cherry tomatoes, halved

1. Preheat the oven to 190°C (fan-forced).
2. Use a small sharp knife to deeply score a diamond pattern into the cut sides of the eggplants, taking care not to cut through the skin.
3. Place the eggplant halves into a large rectangular baking dish (30 cm × 20 cm, approx.), cut sides facing up. Brush the cut surfaces with 2 tablespoons of the olive oil, then spread the crushed garlic over the top. Bake for 25 minutes.
4. Meanwhile, combine the onion, remaining 1 tablespoon of olive oil, balsamic vinegar, tomato paste and sultanas in a bowl and mix well.

5. Top the eggplant halves with the onion mixture and add the tomatoes to the dish. Pour ½ cup (125 ml) water into the baking dish and season with salt and pepper, if desired.

6. Bake for a further 30 minutes, until the eggplant is tender and lightly golden, and the sauce has thickened. Serve immediately.

TZATZIKI – YOGHURT CUCUMBER DIP (with video)

We have served this tzatziki as a dip with fresh veggie sticks, but you could also serve it with some warm bread and olives. Tzatziki is very versatile as it can also be served with grilled fish or lean meat, served with falafel on a wrap, used as a spread on a sandwich, or even as a salad dressing.

Makes 3 cups

Prep Time: 10 minutes

1 large Lebanese cucumber
2 cups (560 g) thick Greek yoghurt
Juice of 1 lemon
1 tablespoon olive oil
1 clove garlic, crushed
Handful of mint leaves, finely chopped (see Note)
Carrot sticks and celery sticks, to serve

1. Grate or finely chop the cucumber into small pieces, including the skin. If you grate the cucumber, squeeze out as much liquid as possible.
2. Place the cucumber into a bowl with the yoghurt, lemon juice, olive oil, garlic and mint. Stir well to combine.
3. Serve with the veggie sticks for dipping. Store in an airtight container in the fridge for up to one week.

Note: You could use dill, chives or parsley instead of mint if that is what you have on hand.

RUSTIC HUMMUS (with video)

Why not try making your own hummus for a change? This Middle
Eastern dip allows the chickpeas to shine, and with the unusual addition
of capers and egg, this is a recipe you will find hard to resist making all
the time.

Makes 1½ cups

Prep Time: 10 minutes
Cooking Time: 7 minutes

Pinch of salt
1 egg
400 g tin chickpeas, rinsed and drained
2 tablespoons tahini
2 cloves garlic, crushed
Juice of ½ large lemon
1 tablespoon capers

1. Half-fill a small saucepan with water and bring to the boil. Add a
   pinch of salt to the boiling water. Using a spoon, gently dip the egg
   in and out of the boiling water, then lower it into the water. This will
   prevent the shell from cracking. Cook for 7 minutes, then remove
   and cool under cold water. Peel the egg and finely chop.
2. Meanwhile, place the chickpeas, tahini, garlic and lemon juice into
   a food processor and process until smooth. Scoop the mixture into
   a bowl and stir in the egg and capers. Season with a little freshly
   ground black pepper if desired.
3. Serve immediately, or store in an airtight container in the fridge for
   up to 5 days.

HOMEMADE BASIL PESTO

Basil is not a difficult herb to grow – it just needs plenty of sun and plenty of water, otherwise it quickly runs to seed. It's a great choice as it's very expensive to buy, and often we only use a little and see the rest go to waste. There is no better feeling than having organic produce at your fingertips, and whenever there's an abundance you can make delicious, nutritious recipes like this.

If you have one, use a mortar and pestle when making this recipe – it gives a rustic finish and taste, and it's a really fun way to make it.

Makes 2 cups

Prep Time: 10 minutes
Cooking Time: 3 minutes

½ cup (80 g) pine nuts (or walnuts)
4 cloves garlic, roughly chopped
½ teaspoon sea salt
½ teaspoon dried chilli flakes
3 cups basil leaves
½ cup (40 g) finely grated parmesan
¼ cup (60 ml) extra virgin olive oil

1. Place the pine nuts into a dry frying pan over medium heat and cook, stirring frequently, for 2–3 minutes until golden. Keep an eye on them as they can burn easily. Transfer to a plate to cool.
2. Using a large mortar and pestle or a food processor, pound or process the garlic, salt and chilli to form a paste.
3. Add the basil and pound or process until a rough puree forms. Add the pine nuts and pound or process using the pulse button, just until they break up a bit (you want a bit of texture here). Add the parmesan and olive oil and combine well.
4. Serve immediately or scoop into an airtight container and keep in the fridge for up to 2 weeks.

QUICK PICKLED ONIONS

These pickled onions are quick and easy to make, and are great to have on hand to add to salads, avocado toast, burrito bowls and more. An empty almond butter or peanut butter jar is perfect to use for this recipe.

Makes 1 jar (375 g)

Prep Time: 10 minutes + at least 1 hour refrigeration
2 red onions, thinly sliced

1 tablespoon honey
Pinch of salt
½ cup (125 ml) white vinegar

1. Wash and sterilise a glass jar (375 g) and its lid (see Note).
2. Place the onions into the glass jar. Squish them down slightly if necessary to fit all of the onion in.
3. Add the honey, salt, vinegar and 1 cup (250 ml) warm water.
4. Secure the lid onto the jar, then gently turn upside down a few times to mix all of the ingredients together.
5. Place the jar into the fridge for at least 1 hour, but they are even better when left in the fridge for a few hours before eating. Keep in the fridge for up to 1 month.

Note: To sterilise the jar, place into a low oven (about 100°C) for 10 minutes, until dry and hot. Remove and cool slightly. Meanwhile, boil the lid in a small saucepan of boiling water for 10 minutes. Remove with tongs and allow to air dry.

MAIN MEALS

BEEF AND ZUCCHINI PIE WITH ROAST VEGGIES

This delicious and nutritious recipe calls for filo pastry, which in contrast to puff pastry has very little saturated fat as it is predominantly water and flour. As with many of the recipes in this book, you shouldn't feel that you have to stick rigidly to the vegetables listed below. It's fine to make substitutions according to what you have on hand.

Serves 6

Prep Time: 20 minutes
Cooking Time: 40 minutes

1 tablespoon olive oil
1 brown onion, finely chopped
500 g lean beef mince
1 carrot, finely chopped
1 potato, peeled and finely chopped
2 zucchini, finely chopped
⅓ cup (40 g) frozen peas
125 g cherry or grape tomatoes, halved
2 tablespoons wholemeal plain flour
1 cup (250 ml) beef or vegetable stock
4–5 sheets filo pastry
Olive oil spray
1 egg, lightly beaten

Roast veggies
2 carrots, cut into bite-sized pieces
1 zucchini, cut into batons
1 sweet potato, peeled and cut into batons
1 potato, peeled and cut into bite-sized pieces
Mixed dried herbs, for sprinkling
1 teaspoon olive oil

1. Heat the olive oil in a large frying pan over medium heat. Add the onion and cook for 4 minutes or until softened and lightly browned. Add the mince and cook, breaking up any lumps with a wooden spoon, until browned.

2. Add the carrot, potato, zucchini, peas and tomatoes. Sprinkle over the flour and cook, stirring, for 1 minute. Stir in the stock and cook for 3–4 minutes or until the vegetables are just tender and the sauce has thickened slightly. Remove from the heat and set aside to cool.

3. Preheat the oven to 200°C (fan-forced). Line a large baking tray with baking paper and spray a large round pie dish (30 cm in diameter, approx.) with olive oil.

4. While the pie filling is cooling, prepare the roast veggies. Toss the vegetables with the herbs and oil to coat. Spread out in a single layer on the prepared baking tray.

5. Lightly spray 3 sheets of pastry with oil and stack together. Use to line the prepared pie dish. Spoon in the cooled filling, then place the remaining pastry sheets (sprayed and stacked) on top. Fold over the overhanging pastry and brush the top with beaten egg.

6. Place the pie and roast veggies in the oven and bake for about 30 minutes, until the pastry is golden and slightly crispy and the vegetables are cooked through. Serve the pie cut into wedges, with the roast veggies on the side.

Note: Instead of making 1 large pie you can make individual pie servings. Spray 1 sheet filo pastry with oil and fold in half to make a square. Use to line a small pie dish, with the edges overhanging. Repeat with the remaining pastry. Place the pie filling into each dish, then gather the overhanging pastry to cover the top of the pies. Brush with beaten egg and bake for 15–20 minutes.

GINGER AND LEMON CHICKEN

A simple chicken meal, perfect for the whole family. Double the recipe and make extra in advance for the week ahead.

Serves 4

Prep Time: 10 minutes
Cooking Time: 10 minutes

2 tablespoons olive oil
4 large chicken thigh fillets, cut into bite-sized pieces
1 teaspoon finely chopped ginger
1 clove garlic, crushed
Finely grated zest and juice of 1 lemon, plus lemon wedges to serve
2 cups (320 g) cooked brown rice, to serve
Flat-leaf parsley leaves, chopped, to serve

1. Heat the oil in a large frying pan over medium-high heat.
2. Add the chicken, ginger and garlic and cook for 5 minutes each side until golden, caramelised and cooked through. Stir the lemon zest and juice through the chicken, then remove from the heat.
3. Serve the chicken with the brown rice, sprinkled with parsley and with lemon wedges on the side.

SPRING GREENS SPAGHETTI

A lovely, fresh pasta dish that makes the most of the delicious seasonal spring vegetables. It's served with cottage cheese, which is high in protein, though you could also serve with grilled chicken breast or chickpeas if you like.

Serves 4

Prep Time: 10 minutes
Cooking Time: 12 minutes

400 g wholemeal spaghetti
1 tablespoon olive oil
2 cloves garlic, crushed
1 bunch asparagus, spears halved
1 cup (120 g) frozen green peas
2 zucchini, cut into thin ribbons (see Note)
Finely grated zest and juice of 1 lemon
Handful of flat-leaf parsley leaves, plus extra to serve
Handful of mint leaves, plus extra to serve
1 cup (200 g) cottage cheese

1. Bring a large saucepan of water to the boil over high heat. Add the spaghetti and cook for about 12 minutes, until al dente (still slightly firm to the bite).
2. When the spaghetti is cooked, reserve 1 cup (250 ml) of the pasta water, then drain. Return the spaghetti to the large saucepan.
3. Meanwhile, heat a small frying pan over medium-low heat. Add the olive oil and garlic and cook for 1–2 minutes, until fragrant. Add the asparagus and cook for 2 minutes, stirring occasionally. Add the frozen peas and cook for a further 2–3 minutes, until thawed and heated through, then remove from the heat.

4. Add the asparagus and pea mixture and the zucchini ribbons to the spaghetti in the large saucepan. Gently stir in the reserved pasta water, lemon zest, juice and herbs until evenly combined.
5. Divide between 4 serving bowls. Top with extra parsley and mint leaves, and serve with a dollop of cottage cheese.

Note: Use a vegetable peeler to cut the zucchini into wide, thin ribbons. Alternatively, thinly slice.

TOFU BANH MI

Banh Mi is a Vietnamese baguette sandwich which often contains pork or ham, so this is a vegetarian version. Tofu is a wonderful staple protein that you can cook in advance and add to your meals throughout the week. It is very versatile as it will soak up whatever flavour you choose to add to it. You could also add some boiled eggs to this recipe, or spice it up with some sliced fresh red chilli.

The tofu in this recipe could also be replaced with chicken.

Serves 4

Prep Time: 15 minutes
Cooking Time: 5 minutes

2 teaspoons canola oil
400 g firm tofu, sliced
4 long crusty wholemeal bread rolls
1 Lebanese cucumber, cut into thin strips
1 carrot, cut into thin matchsticks
1 red capsicum, cut into thin strips
2 tablespoons Quick Pickled Onions (see page 201)
1 tablespoon soy sauce
Juice of 1 lime
Handful of coriander leaves

1. Heat the oil in a large frying pan over medium-high heat. Cook the tofu for about 2 minutes each side, until golden. Transfer to a board to cool slightly, then cut into strips.
2. Cut each of the bread rolls along the centre on top, ensuring not to cut all the way through. Open out the rolls and fill with tofu, cucumber, carrot and capsicum.
3. Add the quick pickled onions, then drizzle with soy sauce and lime juice. Top with coriander leaves and serve immediately.

SPANISH OMELETTE

This is a healthier version of the classic Spanish omelette, which can be served either hot or cold. This can be served as an accompaniment to lunch or dinner, or served with a fresh side salad to make it a meal on its own. It would also be delicious for brunch, served with some sautéed kale and tomatoes.

Serves 4–6

Prep Time: 10 minutes
Cooking Time: 40 minutes

4–5 tablespoons olive oil
5 potatoes, peeled and cut into 5 mm slices
6 large eggs, lightly beaten
Handful of flat-leaf parsley leaves, plus extra to serve

1. Heat the oil in a large non-stick frying pan over medium heat. Add the potato and toss to coat. Reduce the heat to medium-low. Cover the pan and cook the potatoes, turning often, for 20 minutes or until softened slightly.
2. Drain the potatoes in a large colander set over a bowl to catch the oil. Transfer the potatoes to a large bowl and set aside for 5 minutes to cool slightly. Reserve the oil.
3. Gently stir the eggs and parsley into the potato, trying not to break up the slices.
4. Return the frying pan to medium heat and add 3 tablespoons of the reserved oil. Tip the potato mixture into the frying pan and spread out evenly. Cook uncovered for 10 minutes, using a spatula to gently tuck the edges of the omelette into a cushion shape.
5. Once the bottom of the omelette is golden (use a flat-bladed knife to lift an edge slightly to check) and the top is lightly set, carefully invert the omelette onto a large plate.

6. Add 1–2 tablespoons of the reserved oil to the frying pan. Return the omelette to the pan, cooked-side facing up. Cook the omelette for a further 5–10 minutes, tucking in the edges of the omelette again to form the cushion shape, until set and golden brown underneath.

7. Slide the omelette out onto a serving plate. Set aside to cool for 5–10 minutes, then cut into thick wedges. Top with extra parsley to serve.

GRILLED SATAY TOFU

This is a cheat's version of satay tofu – a great shortcut recipe that results in a quick, healthy and delicious meal. When you prepare brown rice, make a large quantity and store it in the fridge for the week. That way it is ready ahead of time, and it is a great addition to meals such as this one. If you are particularly short on time you could substitute for microwave brown rice.

Serves 4

Prep Time: 10 minutes
Cooking Time: 12 minutes

2 tablespoons canola oil
2 bunches bok choy
400 g firm tofu, thickly sliced, then cut into triangles
1 tablespoon curry powder or smoked paprika
⅓ cup (95 g) 100% natural peanut butter
1 tablespoon tamari (or gluten-free soy sauce)
2 cups (320 g) cooked brown rice
Handful of coriander leaves

1. Heat a char-grill pan over medium-high heat. Toss or brush the bok choy with 1 tablespoon of oil. Cook the bok choy for 1–2 minutes on each side, until just charred. Set aside.
2. Place the tofu pieces into a bowl. Sprinkle with the curry powder or paprika and toss to coat.
3. Toss or brush the tofu pieces with the remaining oil. Place the tofu pieces into the pan and cook for 3–4 minutes on each side, until golden and crisp on the surface.
4. Meanwhile, combine the peanut butter, tamari and 1 tablespoon water in a small saucepan. Stir over low heat for about 5 minutes, until heated through.
5. Divide the brown rice between 4 serving bowls. Top with the bok choy and crispy tofu pieces. Drizzle the peanut sauce over the top, then scatter over the coriander leaves. Serve immediately.

MEDITERRANEAN TOFU

A simple Mediterranean-style vegetarian meal. We have served this with wholemeal couscous, but you could serve with pasta or rice if you prefer.

Serves 4

Prep Time: 15 minutes
Cooking Time: 20 minutes

2 cups (400 g) wholemeal couscous
2⅔ cups (660 ml) boiling water
2 tablespoons olive oil
1 red onion, chopped
2 cloves garlic, crushed
2 bunches broccolini, chopped
1 red capsicum, chopped
400 g firm tofu, cut into cubes
2 × 400 g tins crushed tomatoes
½ cup (60 g) pitted black olives
Handful of basil leaves, roughly chopped
Handful of flat-leaf parsley leaves, roughly chopped

1. Place the couscous into a large bowl and pour over the boiling water. Cover tightly and stand for 5–10 minutes, until all the water has been absorbed. Fluff the couscous with a fork to separate the grains, then set aside.
2. Meanwhile, heat the oil in a large saucepan over medium-high heat. Add the onion and garlic and cook, stirring often, for 4–5 minutes until softened. Add the broccolini and capsicum, followed by the tofu. Cook for 5 minutes, stirring occasionally.
3. Stir in the tomatoes and olives and bring to a simmer, then reduce the heat to medium. Cook for 10 minutes, uncovered, until the sauce has thickened.
4. Serve with the couscous, sprinkled with basil and parsley.

MEDITERRANEAN BARRAMUNDI

A flavoursome one-pan fish dish. Barramundi is a great fish to add to your weekly meal plan – keep an eye out for specials and buy in bulk to add to your freezer. Serve with crispy toasted wholegrain bread to mop up the sauce.

Serves 4

Prep Time: 15 minutes
Cooking Time: 20 minutes

2 tablespoons olive oil
1 red onion, chopped
2 cloves garlic, crushed
2 bunches broccolini, chopped
1 red capsicum, chopped
2 × 400 g tins crushed tomatoes
400 g barramundi fillets, skin on, halved
½ cup (60 g) pitted black olives
Handful of basil leaves, roughly chopped
Handful of flat-leaf parsley leaves, roughly chopped

1. Heat the olive oil in a large saucepan over medium-high heat. Add the onion and garlic and cook, stirring often, for 4–5 minutes until softened.
2. Add the broccolini and capsicum, followed by the tomatoes. Stir together and bring to a simmer, then reduce the heat to medium.
3. Add the barramundi and ensure it is covered by the sauce. Add the olives. Cook for 10 minutes, until the fish has turned white and flakes easily when tested with a fork. Remove from the heat.
4. Serve immediately, sprinkled with basil and parsley.

CHILLI CHICKEN STIR-FRY

This is a quick and easy meal to add to your weekly repertoire. It can be whipped up quickly, and you could double the recipe to ensure you have enough leftovers for lunch the next day.

Serves 4

Prep Time: 15 minutes
Cooking Time: 20 minutes

200 g rice vermicelli noodles
2 tablespoons canola oil
1 head broccoli, chopped
1 teaspoon finely grated ginger
1 clove garlic, crushed
400 g chicken mince
2 teaspoons dried chilli flakes
2 tablespoons tamari (or gluten-free soy sauce)
Handful of Thai basil leaves, chopped, to serve
1 lime, quartered, to serve

1. Place the noodles into a large bowl. Cover with boiling water and stand for 5 minutes, until softened. Drain and set aside.
2. Meanwhile, heat 1 tablespoon of the canola oil in a large frying pan over medium-high heat. Add the broccoli and stir-fry for 4–5 minutes, until tender-crisp. Remove from the pan.
3. Heat the remaining oil in the pan. Add the ginger, garlic and then the chicken mince. Cook for 5 minutes, breaking up the mince with a wooden spoon, until lightly browned.
4. Return the cooked broccoli to the pan. Stir in the chilli flakes and tamari and cook for a further 1–2 minutes, until heated through.
5. Divide the vermicelli noodles between 4 serving bowls. Top with the mince mixture and Thai basil leaves. Serve with lime wedges to squeeze over.

PUMPKIN CHICKEN CURRY

This is a great recipe for meal prep – why not double the quantities and make extra to store in the freezer until required? You can get creative with the vegetables that you add in to the curry, as well as the toppings for the curry. Try topping this with some toasted cashews, chopped red chilli, a dollop of yoghurt and some extra fresh coriander.

Serves 4

Prep Time: 15 minutes
Cooking Time: 20 minutes

2 tablespoons canola oil
1 brown onion, chopped
4 chicken thigh fillets, chopped into large pieces
1 teaspoon garam masala
1 teaspoon ground turmeric
1 teaspoon ground cumin
375 ml tin light evaporated milk
½ small butternut pumpkin (about 600 g), peeled, seeded and chopped
1 small eggplant, chopped
1 zucchini, chopped
400 g tin brown lentils, rinsed and drained
1 bunch bok choy, chopped
Handful of coriander leaves
Cooked quinoa, to serve

1. Heat the olive oil in a large saucepan over medium-high heat. Add the onion and chicken. Cook, turning the chicken often, for 4–5 minutes until golden brown. Stir in the garam masala, turmeric and cumin, then pour in the evaporated milk.
2. Add the pumpkin, eggplant and zucchini. Cover and bring to a simmer, then cook for 10 minutes or until the vegetables have softened and the chicken is cooked through.
3. Stir in the lentils, bok choy and coriander. Cook for a further 5 minutes until heated through. Serve with the quinoa.

TOMATO AND BASIL RISONI

Risoni is a wonderful pasta shape for kids, as it cooks quickly and it is small and easy to chew. This is also a one-pot wonder, making it that little bit easier to prepare a meal for the whole family without a lot of washing up!

Serves 4–6

Prep Time: 10 minutes
Cooking Time: 25 minutes

2 tablespoons olive oil
5 Roma tomatoes, chopped
1 red onion, finely chopped
1 clove garlic, crushed
1 cup (220 g) risoni
3 cups (750 ml) vegetable stock (see Note)
2 tablespoons tomato paste
1 cup (120 g) frozen peas
Handful of fresh basil leaves, chopped, plus extra to serve
100 g cherry bocconcini, halved, to serve

1. Heat 1 tablespoon of the oil in a large saucepan over medium-high heat. Add the tomatoes and cook for 4–5 minutes until softened. Remove from the pan and set aside.
2. Heat the remaining oil in the saucepan. Add the onion then the garlic. Cook for 4–5 minutes, stirring often, until the onion is soft.
3. Add the risoni, followed by the stock, and stir briefly. Bring to the boil, then reduce the heat to low. Place a lid on the pan and simmer for 10 minutes, stirring occasionally.

4. Once most of the liquid has been absorbed, stir in the tomato paste and then the frozen peas. Add the cooked tomatoes back into the pan, and cook for a further 5 minutes or until heated through. Remove from the heat and stir in the basil.

5. Serve the risoni topped with the bocconcini and sprinkled with the extra basil.

BEAN AND VEGGIE QUESADILLAS

Your children will love these veggie and cheese filled quesadillas – go ahead and swap the vegetables listed here for what you have on hand, or for what you know your kids will enjoy. These would also be delicious served alongside some homemade guacamole to dip.

Makes 4 (or 8 halves)

Prep Time: 10 minutes
Cooking Time: 20 minutes

1 tablespoon olive oil
½ red onion, thinly sliced
Sprinkle of paprika
Sprinkle of ground cumin
½ × 400 g tin black beans, rinsed and drained
½ × 400 g tin corn kernels, drained
1 tomato, finely chopped
4 wholegrain tortillas or wraps
½ cup (50 g) grated mozzarella

1. Heat the oil in a large frying pan over medium-high heat. Add the onion, paprika and cumin and cook for a couple of minutes, until the onion is starting to soften.
2. Stir in the black beans and corn. Cook for about 4 minutes then stir in the tomato and cook for another minute until the tomato is slightly softened. Transfer the mixture to a bowl and set aside. Give the pan a quick wipe, then return to the heat.
3. Place one tortilla into the pan. Cover half of the tortilla with one-quarter of the bean mixture. Sprinkle one-quarter of the mozzarella over the top. Fold the empty side of the tortilla over the bean filling, and press down to enclose.
4. Cook for about 2 minutes, until lightly toasted underneath. Turn over and cook the other side for about 2 minutes, until lightly golden. Remove from the pan and set aside.
5. Repeat with the remaining ingredients to cook 3 more quesadillas. Cut each one in half to serve.

VEGGIE GNOCCHI BAKE

A great variation on a pasta bake that is a real crowd pleaser. Chop the vegetables finely and this will result in a tomato sauce that is not too chunky, and more palatable to younger children.

Serves 4

Prep Time: 15 minutes
Cooking Time: 45 minutes

2 tablespoons olive oil
1 brown onion, finely chopped
1 carrot, finely chopped
1 stick celery, finely chopped
1 clove garlic, crushed
1 zucchini, finely chopped
1 red capsicum, finely chopped
2 tablespoons tomato paste
500 g packet potato gnocchi
Handful of fresh basil leaves, chopped
⅓ cup (35 g) grated mozzarella

1. Preheat the oven to 190°C (fan-forced). Heat half the oil in a large wide saucepan over medium-high heat. Add the onion, carrot and celery. Cook for 5 minutes or until softened, stirring occasionally. Add the garlic, zucchini and capsicum and continue to cook for a further 5 minutes, stirring occasionally.
2. Mix in the tomato paste then gradually stir in 1½ cups (375 ml) water. Bring to a simmer then reduce the heat to medium. Cook, uncovered, for 10–15 minutes or until vegetables are soft.
3. Meanwhile, heat the remaining oil in a large non-stick frying pan over medium-high heat. Add the gnocchi and cook for 5 minutes, stirring often, until slightly crispy.

4. Remove the tomato sauce from the heat. Add the gnocchi to the tomato sauce, along with the basil leaves, and gently stir to combine. Transfer the mixture to a large round baking dish (approx. 30 cm in diameter). Sprinkle the mozzarella over the top.

5. Bake for 15–20 minutes, until the sauce is bubbling and the cheese is melted and golden. Cool slightly before serving.

PRAWN FRIED RICE (with video)

Black rice is a yummy and healthy variety of rice that is now available in major supermarkets as well as health food stores. Give it a try in this recipe if you have not tried it before. If you can't find it, use brown rice instead. This is an easy and tasty summer meal.

Serves 4

Prep Time: 15 minutes
Cooking Time: 12 minutes

2 tablespoons canola oil
1 carrot, chopped
1 cup (160 g) frozen corn kernels
1 clove garlic, crushed
1 teaspoon finely grated ginger
1 tablespoon gluten-free soy sauce (or tamari)
1 tablespoon gluten-free oyster sauce
1 teaspoon sesame oil
1 cup (200 g) black rice, cooked and cooled
1 cup (120 g) frozen peas
400 g uncooked prawns, peeled and deveined
3 eggs, lightly beaten
Handful of coriander leaves, chopped

1. Heat 1 tablespoon of the oil in a large wok or frying pan over medium-high heat. Add the carrot, corn, garlic and ginger. Cook, stirring often, for 5 minutes until softened.
2. Stir in the soy sauce, oyster sauce and sesame oil. Add the rice and the peas. Cook, stirring often, for 3–4 minutes or until heated through.
3. Meanwhile, heat the remaining oil in a non-stick frying pan over medium-high heat. Add the prawns and cook for 1½ minutes each side, until they have changed colour and are cooked through.

4. Remove the prawns from the pan. Pour in the egg and cook until set. Transfer to a board and chop roughly into small pieces.

5. Top the fried rice with the prawns and egg. Sprinkle with coriander to serve.

PUMPKIN PASTA (with video)

This pasta dish highlights the delicious, sweet flavour of pumpkin.
It might seem unusual to use pumpkin in a pasta dish, but once you
try this recipe you won't question it again!

Serves 6

Prep Time: 10 minutes
Cooking Time: 25 minutes

½ large butternut pumpkin (1 kg), peeled, seeded and chopped (see
    Note)
2 tablespoons olive oil
1 clove garlic, crushed
3 heaped tablespoons tomato paste
1½ cups (375 ml) vegetable stock
½ cup (125 ml) milk
500 g wholemeal pasta (any shape)
400 g tin chickpeas, rinsed and drained
1 bag (60 g) baby spinach
Handful of basil leaves, plus extra to serve

1. Bring a large saucepan of water to the boil over high heat. Add the
   pumpkin and cook for 5–10 minutes until soft. Drain well and set aside.
2. Heat the oil in the same saucepan over medium heat. Add the garlic
   and cook, stirring, for 1 minute or just until fragrant. Add the tomato
   paste and pumpkin and stir to combine. Stir in the stock and milk,
   and season lightly with freshly ground black pepper, if desired.
   Bring to a simmer then cook for a couple of minutes, for the flavours
   to combine.
3. Remove from the heat and use a stick blender to blend the pumpkin
   sauce until thick and smooth. If you would prefer a thinner sauce you
   can add some more water or milk at this step.
4. Meanwhile, bring another large saucepan of water to the boil over
   high heat. Add the pasta and cook for about 12 minutes, until
   al dente (still slightly firm to the bite). Drain the pasta and set aside.

5. Return the pumpkin sauce to the stove over medium heat. Add the chickpeas, baby spinach and basil leaves. Stir well and heat through for 5 minutes.

6. Divide the pasta between serving bowls. Top with the pumpkin sauce and sprinkle with extra basil to serve.

Note: Butternut has a lovely mild, sweet flavour, but you could use any pumpkin variety in season.

FISH PIE

This is a delicious and creamy fish pie – a hearty and wholesome meal for the whole family. You could also make it with filo pastry. Serve with a side of green peas and some steamed green veggies.

Serves 6–8

Prep Time: 15 minutes
Cooking Time: 35 minutes

4 large potatoes, peeled and chopped
2¼ cups (560 ml) milk
2 tablespoons olive oil
1 brown onion, finely chopped
1 carrot, finely chopped
½ cup (60 g) frozen peas and corn mix
2 tablespoons wholemeal plain flour
1 tablespoon wholegrain, Dijon or English mustard
1 cup baby spinach leaves
400 g skinless barramundi fillet (or other white fish) cut into 3 cm pieces
Few sprigs of dill, chopped

1. Preheat the oven to 190°C (fan-forced). Place the potatoes into a large saucepan and cover with water. Bring to the boil over high heat and cook for about 10 minutes, until soft. Drain well and return to the saucepan. Add ¼ cup (60 ml) of the milk and mash until smooth. Set aside.
2. Meanwhile, heat the olive oil in another large saucepan over medium-high heat. Add the onion and carrot and cook, stirring occasionally, for 5 minutes or until softened. Stir in the frozen veggies. Sprinkle the flour over and cook, stirring, for 1 minute.
3. Stir in the mustard, then gradually add the milk, stirring constantly. Bring to a simmer and cook for 4–5 minutes, until thickened. Remove from the heat and gently stir in the baby spinach, fish pieces and dill.

4. Transfer the mixture to a large rectangular baking dish (30 cm × 20 cm, approx.). Top with the mashed potato, and use a fork to create ridges in the surface to help it to crisp up in the oven. If you're using filo pastry to top the pie instead of mash, make sure to glaze the top with a whisked raw egg to help the pastry brown.

5. Bake for 20–25 minutes, until the liquid is bubbling up at the edges and the potato topping is crispy and lightly golden. Cool slightly before serving.

Baby Friendly: Scoop out some of the pie and blend or mash together depending on your child's stage of weaning. Allow to cool before serving.

GREEN MAC 'N' CHEESE

A perfect way to add some extra green veggies into a family favourite meal. This recipe makes a large quantity, and it will last in the fridge for up to 5 days so you might even get a second meal out of it. You can try blending all of the broccoli into the sauce, so that there are no large pieces of broccoli throughout the pasta bake.

Serves 8

Prep Time: 15 minutes
Cooking Time: 45 minutes

600 g pasta elbows
1 head broccoli
2 tablespoons olive oil
1 brown onion, finely chopped
1 leek, finely chopped
1 clove garlic, crushed
1 cup (250 ml) milk
½ cup (40 g) finely grated parmesan

1. Preheat the oven to 180°C (fan-forced). Bring an extra-large pot of water to the boil over high heat. Cut the broccoli into medium florets, then chop the stem. Add the pasta to the boiling water and cook for 4 minutes. Add the broccoli and cook for a further 4–5 minutes, until the pasta is still slightly firm and the broccoli has softened.
2. Reserve 1 cup (250 ml) of the pasta cooking water and set aside. Drain the pasta and broccoli and reserve half the broccoli. Return the pasta and remaining broccoli to the pot.
3. Meanwhile, heat the olive oil in a large saucepan over medium-high heat. Add the onion, leek and garlic. Cook for 5 minutes, stirring often, until soft. Remove from the heat.

4. Add the reserved broccoli, half the reserved pasta water and half the milk to the saucepan with the cooked onion. Use a stick blender to blend everything together until smooth. Gradually add the remaining milk and pasta water and continue to blend until combined into a thick sauce.

5. Pour the green sauce into the pot with the cooked pasta and broccoli. Stir gently until the pasta is coated in the sauce. Transfer to a large rectangular baking dish (30 cm × 20 cm, approx.) and sprinkle with parmesan.

6. Bake for 25 minutes or until crispy and golden on top. Cool slightly before serving.

Baby Friendly: If you are preparing this recipe for a baby, remove a small amount of the green pasta mixture before baking. Blend to a puree or mash the mixture in a bowl, depending on the age of your baby and what weaning stage they are at.

COTTAGE PIE

This is a hearty and wholesome meal for the whole family – there are modifications to make this recipe friendly for infants. Serve the cottage pie with a side of green peas and some steamed green veggies.

Serves 6

Prep Time: 15 minutes
Cooking Time: 1 hour

2 tablespoons olive oil
1 brown onion, finely chopped
1 carrot, finely chopped
1 stick celery, finely chopped
500 g lean beef mince
2 tablespoons wholemeal plain flour
2 tablespoons tomato paste
2 cups (500 ml) beef stock
1 tablespoon Worcestershire sauce
4 potatoes, peeled and chopped
¼ cup (60 ml) milk

1. Preheat the oven to 180°C (fan-forced). Lightly grease a large rectangular baking dish (30 cm × 20 cm, approx.).
2. Heat the olive oil in a large wide saucepan over medium-high heat. Add the onion, carrot and celery. Cook, stirring occasionally, for 5 minutes or until softened. Add the beef mince and cook for a further 5 minutes, breaking up the mince with a wooden spoon, until browned.
3. Sprinkle the flour over and cook, stirring, for 1 minute. Add the tomato paste, stock and Worcestershire sauce and stir to combine. Reduce the heat to medium and simmer for 20 minutes, stirring occasionally, until the liquid has reduced and the sauce has thickened.

4. Meanwhile, place the potatoes into a saucepan. Cover with water and bring to the boil over high heat. Reduce the heat slightly and cook for about 10 minutes, until soft. Drain well and return to the saucepan. Add the milk and mash until smooth.
5. Transfer the beef mixture to the prepared dish. Top with the mashed potato, and use a fork to create ridges in the surface to help it crisp up in the oven.
6. Bake for 20–25 minutes, until the liquid is bubbling up at the edges and the potato topping is crispy and lightly golden. Cool slightly before serving.

Baby Friendly: Remove some of the beef and vegetable mixture at the end of step 2. Allow to cool slightly, then blend or mash depending on your child's weaning stage. You could also add a little of the cooked potato and mash it into the beef mixture.

KID-FRIENDLY TORTELLINI PASTA

Sometimes we need a bit of a shortcut for quick and easy meals. This recipe uses packaged tortellini to put together a meal that is great for busy weeknights. This recipe is simple but tasty, perfect for everyone to enjoy.

Serves 6

Prep Time: 10 minutes
Cooking Time: 15 minutes

600 g packet spinach and cheese tortellini
2 tablespoons olive oil
200 g grape tomatoes, halved
1 red capsicum, chopped
400 g tin butter beans, rinsed and drained
200 g cherry bocconcini, quartered
½ cup basil leaves

1. Bring a large saucepan of water to the boil over high heat. Add the tortellini and cook according to the packet directions, or until al dente (still slightly firm to the bite).
2. Drain the tortellini into a colander and rinse lightly under cold running water. Return the tortellini to the saucepan.
3. Add the olive oil, tomatoes, capsicum, butter beans, bocconcini and basil. Stir to combine. Divide between bowls and serve.

PIZZA BAGELS

You could bump up the veggie content on these bagels if you like – for example with thinly sliced zucchini, mushrooms or roasted pumpkin. This recipe makes for a fun dinner for the whole family – lay out all the ingredients including your chosen vegetable options and allow your children to prepare their own pizza bagels. You could also use up slightly stale bagels in this recipe.

Serves 4

Prep Time: 10 minutes
Cooking Time: 10 minutes

4 wholegrain seeded bagels, halved horizontally
4 tablespoons tomato paste
½ red onion, thinly sliced
1 cup (10 g) grated mozzarella
250 g cherry tomatoes, halved
Flat-leaf parsley and basil leaves, chopped, to serve (optional)

1. Preheat the oven to 200°C (fan-forced). Line 2 baking trays with baking paper.
2. Arrange the bagel halves, cut side up, onto the baking trays. Spread evenly with tomato paste. Top with the onion, mozzarella and tomatoes.
3. Bake for 10 minutes, until the cheese is melted and golden.
4. Sprinkle the fresh herbs over, if using, and serve immediately.

LEMON AND HERB CHICKEN

Prepare this chicken dish in advance to save you time when whipping up a weeknight dinner: make the marinade and then allow the chicken to marinate in the fridge overnight. Serve the chicken with some roasted potatoes and a big leafy green salad.

Serves 4

Prep Time: 5 minutes + marinating time
Cooking Time: 20 minutes

¼ cup (60 ml) olive oil
2 cloves garlic, crushed
Finely grated zest and juice of 1 lemon
2 teaspoons dried oregano
2 teaspoons dried thyme
Sprinkle of paprika
Sprinkle of dried chilli flakes
4 skinless chicken thigh cutlets

1. Whisk all the ingredients (except the chicken) in a large bowl to make a marinade.
2. Add the chicken and turn to coat with the marinade. Cover the bowl and place into the fridge for at least 1 hour (or overnight) to marinate the chicken.
3. Heat a large frying pan or char-grill pan over medium-high heat. Add the chicken and cook for 5–10 minutes on each side, until golden and cooked through.
4. Serve with potatoes and salad, or your chosen accompaniment.

LENTIL MOUSSAKA

Moussaka is a traditional Greek dish consisting of eggplant layered with a rich lamb sauce and topped with a layer of bechamel. This recipe is adapted to a vegetarian version using lentils as the protein source.

Serves 6

Prep Time: 20 minutes
Cooking Time: 55 minutes

2 eggplants, sliced into thin rounds
2 tablespoons olive oil
1 clove garlic, crushed
1 brown onion, finely chopped
1 red capsicum, finely chopped
2 tablespoons tomato paste
2 × 400 g tins cherry tomatoes
2 × 400 g tins brown lentils, rinsed and drained
1 cup (200 g) smooth ricotta
2 eggs
1 cup (280 g) Greek yoghurt
Sprinkle of nutmeg
½ cup (40 g) finely grated parmesan

1. Preheat the oven to 180°C (fan-forced). Heat a large non-stick frying pan over medium heat. Cook the eggplant in batches for 2 minutes each side until slightly softened, then transfer to a plate and set aside. (You don't need oil here – it is just to soften the eggplant.)
2. Heat a large saucepan over medium heat. Add the olive oil and garlic and cook for a couple of minutes, until fragrant. Add the onion and capsicum and cook for 3–4 minutes, until starting to soften. Stir in the tomato paste, tomatoes and lentils. Cook for 10 minutes, uncovered, until the sauce has thickened slightly.
3. Meanwhile, to prepare the topping, whisk the ricotta, eggs and yoghurt in a bowl until smooth. Add the nutmeg and season with freshly ground black pepper if desired. Whisk to combine, then set aside.

4. Spread a small amount of the lentil sauce over the base of a rectangular baking dish (30 cm × 20 cm, approx.). Top with one-third of the eggplant slices, overlapping them slightly to form a neat layer. Top with one-third of the lentil sauce. Continue with the remaining eggplant and lentil sauce to make two more layers of each.

5. Dollop the ricotta mixture over the top of the lentil sauce and spread out as evenly as possible. Sprinkle the parmesan over the top.

6. Bake for 25–30 minutes, until the sauce is bubbling around the edges of the dish and the topping is set and golden brown. Set aside for 5 minutes before serving.

Note: The moussaka will be even better if made the day before serving – this will allow it extra time to sit and absorb the flavours, and the eggplant layers will hold together better when slicing. Store in the fridge for 1 day, then slice and reheat in the oven or microwave before serving.

ONE-PAN SICILIAN CHICKEN

This dish is inspired by the flavours of Sicily – Italy's small southern island. In Sicily this dish would be prepared with swordfish as the protein source, however we have swapped it here for chicken as it is more accessible in Australia. If you can find steaks of swordfish at your local fishmonger, give it a try! This is great with some cooked green beans and a fresh rocket salad.

Serves 4

Prep Time: 10 minutes
Cooking Time: 50 minutes

¼ cup (60 ml) olive oil
2 cloves garlic, finely chopped
8 chicken drumsticks
250 g cherry tomatoes, halved
1 long red chilli, seeds removed, chopped
½ cup (60 g) pitted black olives
2 tablespoons capers
2 cups (500 ml) chicken stock

1. Heat the oil in a large non-stick frying pan or cast iron pan over medium heat. Add the garlic and cook for a couple of minutes, until fragrant.
2. Add the chicken and cook for about 5 minutes, turning as needed, until evenly browned. Add the cherry tomatoes, chilli, olives and capers to the pan.
3. Pour in a small amount of the stock and stir gently to deglaze the pan, then add the remaining stock. Bring to a simmer, then reduce the heat to low and cover the pan with a lid. Cook for 20 minutes.
4. Increase the heat to medium and remove the lid. Turn the chicken and cook for a further 20 minutes, until some of the liquid has evaporated and the chicken is cooked through. Serve with sides of your choice.

Note: Deglazing the pan means you use a little liquid (in this case the stock) to dislodge and lift the brown bits from frying off the base of the pan, so they mix through the sauce and add lots of flavour.

GREEK CHICKEN GYROS

A healthier take on the popular Greek fast food. This one is made with lean grilled chicken and packed full of flavoursome favourites such as Greek salad and tzatziki. Begin this recipe a few hours ahead, to allow time for the chicken to marinate.

Serves 4

Prep Time: 10 minutes + marinating time
Cooking Time: 10 minutes

2 tablespoons olive oil
1 tablespoon lemon juice
1 clove garlic, crushed
¼ cup (70 g) Greek yoghurt
1 teaspoon dried oregano
1 teaspoon ground cumin
400 g chicken thigh fillets, excess fat removed
8 small pita breads or flat breads
1½ cups (375 ml) Tzatziki (see page 198)
Greek Salad (see page 181)

1. Place 1 tablespoon of the oil, the lemon juice, garlic, yoghurt, oregano and cumin into a large bowl and mix until well combined. Add the chicken and mix to coat with the marinade. Cover and place into the fridge for 3–4 hours to marinate.
2. To cook the chicken, heat the remaining oil in a large non-stick frying pan over medium-high heat. Add the chicken and cook for 3–4 minutes on each side, until browned and cooked through. Transfer the chicken to a board and cool slightly before cutting into thick slices.
4. Meanwhile, warm the pita breads in the microwave for 30 seconds (if desired). Place two pita breads each onto four serving plates.
5. Spread each pita bread with a tablespoon of tzatziki. Top with the Greek salad and the sliced chicken. Drizzle with the remaining tzatziki and serve immediately.

EASY NO-BAKE NACHOS (with video)

A quick and easy meal to serve for lunch or dinner. You can even prepare the tomato and bean sauce in advance, then reheat when you are ready to serve. Serve with a fresh tomato salsa or other chopped fresh veggies, and some sliced jalapenos, depending on the age of your children.

Serves 4

Prep Time: 10 minutes
Cooking Time: 20 minutes

2 tablespoons olive oil
1 brown onion, chopped
1 clove garlic, crushed
Sprinkle of paprika
400 g tin black beans, rinsed and drained
400 g tin red kidney beans, rinsed and drained
400 g tin cherry tomatoes
300 g packet plain low-salt corn chips
1 avocado, diced
Chopped coriander leaves and Greek yoghurt, to serve

1. Heat the olive oil in a large saucepan over medium heat. Add the onion, garlic and paprika. Cook for about 5 minutes, stirring occasionally, until the onion is soft.
2. Add the black beans, red kidney beans, cherry tomatoes and ½ cup (125 ml) water. Season with freshly ground black pepper if desired, and stir to combine.
3. Bring to a simmer, then reduce the heat to low. Cook for 15 minutes, stirring occasionally, until thickened.
4. Arrange the corn chips into 4 shallow serving bowls. Spoon the bean mixture onto the corn chips, then top with the avocado, coriander and a dollop of Greek yoghurt. Serve immediately.

CHICKPEA GYROS

Inspired by Greek gyros, this is a healthier vegetarian option. Packed full of Greek flavours such as Greek salad and tzatziki, these wraps are bursting with flavour and nourishing ingredients. These are best enjoyed right away.

Serves 4

Prep Time: 10 minutes
Cooking Time: 10 minutes

2 tablespoons olive oil
2 × 400 g tins chickpeas, rinsed and drained
Large pinch of dried oregano
8 small pita breads or flat breads
1½ cups (375 ml) Tzatziki (see page 198)
16 cos lettuce leaves
Greek Salad (see page 181)

1. Heat the oil in a non-stick frying pan over medium heat. Add the chickpeas and oregano, and toss to coat.
2. Fry the chickpeas for about 10 minutes, stirring often, until they are lightly golden and crispy. Remove from the heat.
3. Meanwhile, warm the pita breads in the microwave for 30 seconds (if desired). Place two pita breads each onto four serving plates.
4. Spread each pita bread with a tablespoon of tzatziki. Top with the lettuce, Greek salad and the crispy chickpeas. Drizzle with the remaining tzatziki and serve immediately.

CAULIFLOWER FRIED RICE

This is a flavoursome and speedy recipe. If you would like to bump up the protein you could add an extra tin of lentils, toss some fried eggs through, or grill some lean meat to serve on the side. This recipe is a great way to use up any extra rice that you have left over in your fridge. Using rice that was boiled the day before and stored in the fridge will produce the best fluffy fried rice.

Serves 4

Prep Time: 15 minutes
Cooking Time: 25 minutes

2 tablespoons canola oil
1 brown onion, sliced
1 clove garlic, crushed
1 teaspoon finely grated ginger
1 cauliflower, cut into small florets
1 red capsicum, chopped
1 teaspoon ground turmeric
1 tablespoon curry powder
120 g haloumi, cut into small cubes
400 g tin brown lentils, rinsed and drained
2 cups (320 g) cooked brown basmati rice
1 tablespoon chilli paste or 1 thinly sliced red chilli
1 bag (60 g) baby spinach leaves
Handful of coriander leaves

1. Heat a large wok over medium-high heat. Add the canola oil and onion. Cook for 1–2 minutes, until just soft, then add the garlic, ginger and cauliflower. Cook for 5 minutes, stirring often.
2. Add the capsicum, turmeric and curry powder and stir through, ensuring the vegetables are coated with the spices. Cook for a further 5 minutes, until the cauliflower is soft.

3. Push the vegetables to one side of the wok to make some space, then fry the haloumi for 1–2 minutes, until lightly golden.

4. Add the lentils and rice to the wok. Turn the heat up to high and stir to combine all of the ingredients. Cook for 5 minutes, stirring often.

5. Reduce the heat to medium and add in the chilli paste, baby spinach and coriander. Toss to combine. Cook for a further 3–4 minutes, stirring often to ensure everything is coated in the spices and chilli paste. Serve immediately.

BAKED BEANS (with video)

This is a simple and versatile dish that can be put together in minutes. It's perfect for a satisfying meal at any time of day. Why not double the recipe and store in the fridge for up to 5 days – great for a last-minute meal, or to have as a snack. If you like, add a sprinkle of chilli flakes to spice things up!

Serves 4

Prep Time: 5 minutes
Cooking Time: 25 minutes

1 tablespoon olive oil
½ red onion, diced
½ large carrot, diced
1 stick celery, diced
400 g tin crushed tomatoes
400 g tin cannellini beans, rinsed and drained

1. Heat the olive oil in a large saucepan over medium heat. .
2. Add the onion, carrot and celery. Cook for about 10 minutes, stirring often, until soft and golden. You want to release all the natural sweetness in the vegetables so that you don't have to add any sugar.
3. Add the tomatoes. Swish ½ cup (125 ml) water in the can to rinse any remaining tomato and add to the pan. Cook over medium-low heat for about 10 minutes, until the liquid has reduced and the mixture has thickened slightly.
4. Stir in the beans and cook for a few minutes, to heat through. Season with some pepper, if desired.

VIETNAMESE-STYLE VERMICELLI SALAD BOWL (with video)

A fresh and flavoursome dish – delicious served warm right away or packed as a cold lunch during the week. This version uses tofu and egg as the protein source, but you could just as easily use minute steak, chicken or fish. You could also add extra veggies such as capsicum, broccoli, cabbage or cauliflower.

Serves 4

Prep Time: 15 minutes
Cooking Time: 10 minutes

200 g rice vermicelli noodles
400 g firm tofu, cut into thin strips
1 tablespoon canola oil
4 eggs
2 large carrots, cut into thin strips
2 large celery sticks, cut into thin strips
250 g cherry tomatoes, halved
1 cup (80 g) beansprouts
¼ cup (35 g) unsalted roasted peanuts, chopped

Dressing
2 tablespoons soy sauce
1 tablespoon fish sauce
1 tablespoon honey
1 teaspoon sesame oil
1 clove garlic, crushed
Sprinkle of dried chilli flakes, plus extra to serve

1. Place the noodles into a large bowl. Cover with boiling water and stand for 5 minutes, until softened. Drain and set aside.
2. To prepare the dressing, place the ingredients into a jar. Tighten the lid then shake well to combine. Set aside until needed.
3. Heat a non-stick frying pan over medium heat. Add the tofu strips with 1 tablespoon canola oil and fry for 10 minutes, turning as needed, until golden and crisp on the outside. Remove from the pan.

4. Return the pan to low heat. Crack the eggs into the pan and cook, covered, for 3–4 minutes until done to your liking.

5. Place the vermicelli into a large mixing bowl. Add the carrot, celery and tomatoes. Toss to combine. Pour the dressing over the salad and toss to coat.

6. Divide the salad between 4 serving bowls. Top each bowl with the tofu, beansprouts, a fried egg, chilli flakes and peanuts. Serve immediately.

STUFFED MUSHROOMS (with video)

These mushrooms are delicious as a main meal served with roast vegetables or a salad. Feel free to substitute the vegetables for any others you already have in your fridge. You could also add some cooked brown rice or quinoa if you have leftovers.

Serves 4

Prep Time: 15 minutes
Cooking Time: 35 minutes

3 teaspoons olive oil (or oil from the sun-dried tomato jar)
1 small brown onion, diced
2 cloves garlic, crushed
1 zucchini, diced
1 yellow capsicum, chopped
1 tablespoon sun-dried tomatoes, chopped
1 tablespoon pitted black olives, chopped
4 large portobello mushrooms, stalks removed and chopped
Large sprinkle of dried oregano
Large sprinkle of dried chilli flakes
2 tablespoons grated cheddar cheese

1. Preheat the oven to 180°C (fan-forced). Heat the oil in a non-stick frying pan over medium heat. Add the onion and garlic and cook for about 5 minutes, stirring occasionally, until softened.
2. Add the zucchini, capsicum, sun-dried tomatoes, olives and mushroom stalks. Stir in the oregano and chilli flakes. Cook for 10 minutes, stirring occasionally, until soft. Remove from the heat.
3. Arrange mushrooms top-side down on a baking tray. Divide the vegetable mixture evenly between the mushrooms. Sprinkle with cheese.
4. Bake for 15–20 minutes, until the mushrooms are soft and the cheese is melted and lightly golden. Serve immediately.

EGGPLANT LASAGNE

A flavoursome vegetarian version of lasagne. This recipe mainly requires some pantry staples, meaning you can make it quite cheaply. If eggplant is not in season, try zucchini instead, cut into thick long slices.

Serves 6

Prep Time: 15 minutes
Cooking Time: 55 minutes

1 tablespoon olive oil
1 clove garlic, crushed
2 × 400 g tins whole tomatoes
500 ml tomato passata
1 small bunch basil, leaves picked
2 large eggplants, sliced into thin rounds
300 g dried lasagne sheets
¾ cup (150 g) smooth ricotta
½ cup (50 g) grated mozzarella

1. Preheat the oven to 180°C (fan-forced). Heat a large saucepan over medium heat. Add the olive oil and garlic, and cook for a couple of minutes until fragrant.
2. Add the tomatoes and tomato passata. Stir in ½ cup (125ml) water. Use a large spoon to break up the whole tomatoes. Bring just to the boil then reduce the heat to low. Add the basil leaves and simmer for 5–10 minutes until the sauce reduces slightly, then remove from the heat.
3. Meanwhile, heat a large non-stick frying pan over medium heat. Cook the eggplant in batches for 2 minutes each side until lightly browned and softened. (You don't need oil here – it is just to soften the eggplant.) Set aside.

4. Spread a thin layer of the tomato sauce over the base of a large rectangular baking dish (30 cm × 20 cm, approx.). Add a single layer of lasagne sheets, then cover with a thin layer of the tomato sauce. Add a single layer of the fried eggplant, followed by a few dollops of the ricotta. Cover this with another single layer of lasagne sheets, tomato sauce, eggplant and ricotta.

5. Continue layering, finishing with lasagne sheets covered in a thicker layer of the remaining tomato sauce. Sprinkle with the mozzarella.

6. Bake for 35–40 minutes, until the sauce is bubbling, the pasta is tender and the cheese is golden. Check towards the end of cooking time, and if the top starts to look too dark you can cover with foil for the last part.

7. Set aside to rest and cool slightly for 5–10 minutes before cutting into portions. Serve with a side salad.

Tip: The lasagne will be even better if made in advance the day before serving – this will allow it extra time to sit and develop the flavours, and the layers will hold together better when slicing. Store the lasagne in the fridge, then slice and reheat in the oven or microwave before serving.

CHICKEN SUSHI BOWL

A simple lunch or dinner meal that can be thrown together with leftovers. This is also a good meal to prep in advance and store in the freezer for weekday lunches. You could also add some edamame, very thinly sliced carrots, seaweed salad – get creative!

Serves 4

Prep Time: 10 minutes

1⅓ cups (180 g) cooked basmati rice
2 tablespoons rice vinegar
2 cooked chicken breast fillets, chopped
2 small Lebanese cucumbers, chopped
2 small avocados, sliced
4 nori sheets
Reduced-salt gluten-free soy sauce (or tamari), dried chilli flakes and
    pickled ginger, to serve (optional)

1. Reheat the rice in a medium bowl in the microwave. Add the rice vinegar and use a metal spoon to fold through until combined.
2. Divide the rice between 4 serving bowls. Top with the chicken, cucumber and avocado. Fold the nori sheets in half and arrange at the edge of the bowls.
3. Serve with soy sauce, chilli flakes and pickled ginger, if using.

BAKED GREEN CURRY CAULIFLOWER

A simple dish suitable for a weeknight dinner – just place everything in a dish and into the oven, put the rice on to cook and get on with other tasks. This dish would also work well served with a dollop of yoghurt to cut through the spice of the curry paste.

Serves 4

Prep Time: 10 minutes
Cooking Time: 45 minutes

½ large cauliflower, chopped into florets
1 brown onion, chopped
400 g tin chickpeas, rinsed and drained
1–2 tablespoons green curry paste
400 g tofu, cubed (see Note)
1 cup (200 g) brown rice
4 spring onions, sliced

1. Preheat the oven to 200°C (fan-forced). Place the cauliflower, onion and chickpeas into a large baking dish (30 cm × 20 cm, approx.). Dollop the green curry paste over. Stir well to make sure everything is coated in the curry paste. Top with the tofu.
2. Bake for 20 minutes. Remove from the oven and give everything a stir. Return to the oven for a further 20–25 minutes, until the tofu is lightly golden and the cauliflower is cooked through.
3. Meanwhile, cook the brown rice in a large saucepan of boiling water for 30 minutes or until tender.
4. Top the baked curry with the spring onions. Serve immediately, with a side of brown rice.

Note: If you prefer (and dairy isn't a problem), replace the tofu with cubed paneer. This is a cheese which is similar to feta, though not as salty, and is used in Indian cuisine.

CAULIFLOWER AND BLACK BEAN TACOS

These vegan tacos are quick and easy to whip up for a weeknight dinner. You can get creative and add extra toppings or accompaniments to these tacos, such as a fresh tomato salsa, some charred corn or roasted capsicum.

Serves 4

Prep Time: 10 minutes
Cooking Time: 25 minutes

1 head cauliflower, chopped into florets
¼ cup (60 ml) olive oil
1 teaspoon ground cumin
1 teaspoon paprika
1 teaspoon chilli powder
1 teaspoon garlic powder
8 small corn tortillas
1 large avocado, lightly mashed
400 g tin black beans, rinsed and drained
½ red cabbage, thinly sliced
2 tomatoes, diced
Handful of fresh coriander leaves
2 radishes, thinly sliced
1 lime, cut into wedges

1. Preheat the oven to 180°C (fan-forced). Arrange the cauliflower florets over 2 baking trays. Drizzle with the olive oil and sprinkle with the cumin, paprika, chilli powder and garlic powder. Roast for 20 minutes, until tender and golden. Set aside.
2. Place the tortillas, wrapped in foil, into the oven to heat through for 5 minutes.
3. To assemble, spread a small amount of avocado onto each tortilla. Top with the roasted cauliflower, black beans, cabbage, tomatoes, coriander and radish.
4. Serve immediately, with lime wedges to squeeze over.

FETA PASTA (with video)

This recipe is simple and can be whipped up easily on a weeknight. Why not try experimenting by adding different veggies in with the roast tomatoes? Try red onion, capsicum, olives or whatever is in the fridge. Serve with pine nuts, chilli flakes and cracked black pepper, if desired.

Serves 4–5

Prep Time: 10 minutes
Cooking Time: 35 minutes

200 g reduced-fat feta
500 g large truss tomatoes, chopped
200 g grape tomatoes
Drizzle of olive oil
2 tablespoons balsamic vinegar
3 cloves garlic, peeled
Sprinkle of dried oregano
2 large zucchini
250 g wholemeal spaghetti
Handful of basil or flat-leaf parsley leaves

1. Preheat the oven to 200°C (fan-forced). Place the feta in the centre of a large baking dish (30 cm × 20 cm, approx.). Arrange the tomatoes around the feta. Drizzle with olive oil and the balsamic vinegar. Add the whole garlic cloves and sprinkle with dried oregano. Roast for 30–35 minutes, until the feta is golden and the tomatoes are blistered.
2. Meanwhile, use a spiraliser, or vegetable or julienne peeler to cut the zucchini into long spaghetti-like strips. Set aside.
3. Bring a medium saucepan of water to the boil over high heat. Add the spaghetti and cook for about 12 minutes, until al dente (still slightly firm to the bite). Reserve ½ cup (125 ml) of the pasta water then drain the spaghetti.

4. Use a fork to mash the roasted feta, tomatoes and garlic together. It may not look appetising at this point, but it will all come together to form the pasta sauce.
5. Add the zucchini and spaghetti to the baking dish. Use tongs to gently combine with the sauce, adding a dash of the reserved pasta water to bring it all together.
6. Sprinkle with the basil or parsley and serve immediately.

PRAWN AND MANGO TACOS

Celebrate summer mango season with this delicious taco dish.
You could also try cooking the prawns on the barbecue instead.

Serves 4

Prep Time: 15 minutes
Cooking Time: 5 minutes

10 cherry tomatoes, chopped
1 Lebanese cucumber, diced
1 small mango, diced
1 avocado, diced
¼ red onion, diced
½ cup coriander leaves, plus extra to serve
1 lime, halved, plus wedges to serve
1 teaspoon olive oil
1 clove garlic
400 g uncooked prawns, peeled
½ teaspoon paprika
8 mini wholemeal tortillas, heated if desired

1. Combine the tomato, cucumber, mango, avocado, onion and
   coriander in a small bowl. Squeeze the lime juice over and stir
   through. Set aside.
2. Heat the olive oil in a small frying pan over medium heat. Add the
   garlic and cook for 1 minute, until fragrant. Add the prawns and
   paprika. Cook, tossing occasionally, for 4–5 minutes until the prawns
   change colour and are cooked through.
3. Fill the tortillas with the mango mixture and the cooked prawns.
   Sprinkle over some more coriander and serve with lime wedges.

SUPER VEG SPAGHETTI

A hearty vegetarian pasta dish that is easy to prepare. This dish is designed for you to be able to substitute with whatever vegetables you have in your fridge. The lentils add protein to this dish which will fill you up, and they can be substituted with another legume such as chickpeas or red kidney beans.

Serves 4

Prep Time: 10 minutes
Cooking Time: 20 minutes

400 g wholemeal spaghetti
1 tablespoon garlic-infused olive oil (see Note)
1 brown onion, chopped
1 teaspoon dried oregano
1 carrot, chopped
1 zucchini, chopped
½ bunch kale, chopped
1 red capsicum, chopped
400 g tin crushed tomatoes
400 g tin brown lentils, rinsed and drained
Basil leaves, chopped, to serve

1. Bring a large saucepan of water to the boil over high heat. Add the spaghetti and cook for about 12 minutes, until al dente (still slightly firm to the bite).
2. Meanwhile, heat the oil in a saucepan over medium heat. Add the onion and oregano and cook for 5 minutes. Add the carrot and zucchini and cook for another 3–4 minutes, until starting to soften. Stir in the kale and capsicum.
3. Add the tomatoes and lentils. Bring to the boil and cook for 5–10 minutes, until the sauce has reduced and thickened. Season with freshly ground black pepper to taste.
4. Drain the pasta and divide between 4 bowls. Top with the vegetable sauce and a sprinkle of basil. Serve immediately.

Note: You can use olive oil and 1 crushed garlic clove instead if you like.

ZUCCHINI AND CHICKPEA FRITTERS

Fritters are an underrated dish as they are simple to prepare, can be cooked in large batches and then stored in the fridge or freezer for future meals, and they taste delightful! These fritters work well served with a side salad, or on a wholemeal bun as a burger.

Serves 4 (Makes 25 small or 12 large fritters)

Prep Time: 10 minutes
Cooking Time: 20 minutes

400 g tin chickpeas, rinsed and drained
4 small zucchini
3 eggs, lightly beaten
150 g feta, crumbled
¾ cup (120 g) wholemeal plain flour
1 teaspoon baking powder
½ cup basil leaves, chopped
½ cup flat-leaf parsley leaves, chopped
olive oil, to fry

1. Place the chickpeas into a large mixing bowl and use a fork to mash them (they won't be perfectly smooth). Grate the zucchini and squeeze out the excess water. Stir into the chickpeas.
2. Add the eggs, feta, flour, baking powder, basil and parsley. Season with pepper to taste. Mix well to combine all the ingredients.
3. Heat a small amount of olive oil in a large non-stick frying pan over medium-high heat. Add heaped tablespoons of the mixture to the pan and flatten out. Cook for 3 minutes each side until golden and cooked through. Transfer to a tray lined with paper towel.
4. Continue to cook fritters in batches, adding a small amount of olive oil each time, until all the fritter mixture has been used.
5. Serve fritters with a side salad, or on a bun.

CAULIFLOWER MARGHERITA PIZZAS

Using cauliflower to make the bases for this pizza is a surprisingly delicious way to include some more vegetables into your meal. Once you have mastered the pizza base recipe you can top it with unlimited combinations of vegetables, herbs and spices.

Serves 4

Prep Time: 20 minutes
Cooking Time: 40 minutes

1 head cauliflower, leaves removed, roughly chopped
¾ cup (90 g) ground almonds
3 eggs
1 teaspoon garlic powder
4 tablespoons tomato paste
2 large tomatoes, diced (see Note)
150 g cherry bocconcini, sliced
Handful of basil leaves, plus extra to serve

1. Preheat the oven to 200°C (fan-forced). Line 2 large baking trays with baking paper.
2. Working in batches, process the cauliflower in a food processor to the texture of coarse breadcrumbs. Transfer to a mixing bowl and add the ground almonds, eggs and garlic powder. Season lightly with salt and freshly ground black pepper if desired. Mix well until combined and the mixture resembles a dough.
3. Divide into 4 portions. Spread onto the baking trays, shaping into rough circles that are 20 cm in diameter. Make sure the thickness is even. Place the pizza bases into the oven and bake for 20–30 minutes, until golden and crispy around the edges.

4. Set aside to cool slightly. Slide a large knife under the bases to loosen from the baking paper. Spread the tomato paste over the bases and top with the remaining ingredients.

5. Bake for 5–10 minutes, until the cheese is melted. Top with extra basil leaves and serve.

Note: Use 500 g halved cherry tomatoes in place of large tomatoes, if you prefer.

SALMON QUICHE WITH ALMOND PASTRY

This recipe takes slightly more time and effort than our usual recipes on this program, so it is perfect for a weekend lunch or dinner, or to make ahead and take to a friend's place for a meal. The result is worth the extra effort!

Serves 8

Prep Time: 15 minutes
Cooking Time: 50 minutes

2½ cups (300 g) ground almonds
8 eggs
1 tablespoon olive oil
Pinch of freshly ground black pepper
½ cup (125 ml) milk
1 zucchini, thinly sliced
1 small red onion, thinly sliced
Handful of baby spinach leaves
210 g tin red salmon, drained and coarsely flaked
1 tablespoon chopped dill

1. Preheat oven to 180°C (fan-forced). Place a round 30 cm tart tin onto a baking tray and set aside.
2. To make the almond pastry, combine the ground almonds, 2 eggs, the olive oil and the black pepper in a mixing bowl. Stir until the mixture comes together and forms a dough.
3. Place the dough between 2 sheets of baking paper. Use a rolling pin to roll the pastry into a large circle (36 cm). Peel the top layer of paper from the dough. Invert over the tart tin and peel off the remaining paper. Carefully press the dough into the base and sides of the tin. If any holes form, you can use your fingers to mould the dough back together.
4. Keep the tart tin on the baking tray to make it easier to remove from the oven. Bake for 15–20 minutes, until light golden brown.

5. Meanwhile, for the filling, whisk the remaining 6 eggs with the milk. Add the zucchini, onion, baby spinach, salmon and dill. Season with freshly ground black pepper if desired.

6. Pour the filling mixture into the pastry case. Spread with a spoon to make sure the salmon and vegetables are evenly distributed.

7. Bake for 20–30 minutes, until the egg mixture is set in the middle. Cool slightly, then cut into wedges to serve.

HEALTHIER PAD THAI

A healthier version of a takeaway favourite because it has more veggies! You can also substitute the vegetables for any that you already have at home. Tamarind paste should be available from any large supermarket, or Asian grocer.

Serves 4

Prep Time: 20 minutes
Cooking Time: 15 minutes

250 g rice stick noodles
1 tablespoon canola oil
1 clove garlic, crushed
1 teaspoon finely grated ginger
300 g firm tofu, cut into bite-sized pieces
1 tablespoon gluten-free soy sauce (or tamari)
Sprinkle of dried chilli flakes
1 carrot, thinly sliced
1 red capsicum, thinly sliced
3 spring onions, sliced
2 large kale leaves, torn
3 eggs, lightly whisked
1 cup (80 g) bean sprouts
Handful of coriander leaves
¼ cup (35 g) unsalted roasted peanuts, roughly chopped
Lime wedges, to serve

Sauce
2 tablespoons tamarind paste
2 tablespoons gluten-free soy sauce (or tamari)
1 tablespoon sriracha
2 tablespoons lime juice

1. Place the noodles into a large bowl and cover with boiling water. Soak for 6 minutes until soft. Drain and set aside. Combine the sauce ingredients in a small bowl.
2. Heat a large non-stick frying pan over medium heat. Add the oil, garlic and ginger and cook for 1 minute, until fragrant. Add the tofu, soy sauce and chilli flakes and cook for a couple of minutes on each side, until browned.
3. Transfer the tofu to a plate and set aside. Add the vegetables to the pan. Str-fry for 5 minutes, until softened.
4. Push the vegetables to one side of the pan, then pour the eggs into the empty space. Cook for a couple of minutes, until just set, then stir the vegetables back through. Add the noodles and tofu. Drizzle with the sauce and toss gently to combine and to ensure that everything is coated and heated through.
5. Divide the Pad Thai between 4 bowls. Top with the bean sprouts, coriander and peanuts. Serve with lime wedges to squeeze over.

MAPLE TOFU STIR-FRY

You will love tofu once you give this recipe a try! The sauce is slightly sweet and slightly salty, and the crisp texture of the fried tofu is delicious. As always, you could substitute whatever vegetables are in your fridge!

Serves 4

Prep Time: 15 minutes
Cooking Time: 25 minutes

1 cup (200 g) brown rice
1 tablespoon canola oil
400 g firm tofu, cut into cubes
½ head broccoli, chopped into small pieces (stem included)
1 large zucchini, chopped
4 spring onions, sliced, plus extra to serve
Sesame seeds, to serve
Dried chilli flakes, to serve

Sauce
2 tablespoons pure maple syrup (not maple-flavoured syrup)
2 tablespoons gluten-free soy sauce (or tamari)
1 tablespoon red wine vinegar
1 tablespoon finely grated ginger

1. Place the brown rice into a medium saucepan with 2 cups (500 ml) water and bring to the boil. Once boiling, cover and reduce the heat to low then simmer for 30 minutes or until all the water is absorbed and the rice is tender.
2. Meanwhile, heat the oil in a large frying pan over medium-high heat. Add the tofu and cook for 2 minutes on one side until it is very golden and crisp. Turn over and cook for another 2 minutes on the other side.

3. Push the tofu to one side of the pan to continue cooking the other sides of the cubes. Add the broccoli, zucchini and spring onions. Cook, stirring for 3–5 minutes, until the vegetables are just tender.

4. Combine the sauce ingredients in a small bowl. Pour the sauce over the vegetables and tofu and stir-fry for another minute, until the sauce has thickened slightly. Remove from the heat.

5. Divide the rice between 4 bowls. Top with the tofu and vegetable mixture. Sprinkle with extra spring onion, sesame seeds and chilli flakes to serve.

HEARTY VEGETARIAN SHEPHERD'S PIE

This lentil and vegetable-based shepherd's pie is so rich and flavoursome, you won't even notice that it doesn't contain meat. The garlic potato mash on top makes it even more delicious. This recipe is best suited to a weekend when you can spend a bit of extra time cooking.

Serves 10

Prep Time: 25 minutes
Cooking Time: 1 hour

1 bulb fennel, cut into small pieces
1 parsnip, cut into small pieces
3 carrots, cut into small pieces
1 tablespoon olive oil
1 teaspoon chopped rosemary
1 teaspoon ground nutmeg

Sauce
1 tablespoon olive oil
1 brown onion, sliced
1 teaspoon dried thyme
1 teaspoon dried oregano
1 cup (250 ml) vegetable stock
2 tablespoons balsamic vinegar
400g tin brown lentils, rinsed and drained
500 ml passata

Topping
6 large potatoes, peeled and cut into small cubes
2 cloves garlic, peeled
2 tablespoons olive oil

1. Preheat the oven to 180°C (fan-forced). Line a large baking tray with baking paper. Place the fennel, parsnip and carrot onto the tray. Drizzle with the olive oil and sprinkle with the rosemary and nutmeg. Mix everything together then spread the vegetables out evenly on the tray. Bake for 15 minutes, then turn the vegetables over and return to the oven for a further 10 minutes.

2. Meanwhile, to make the sauce, heat the oil in a large saucepan over medium heat. Add the onion, thyme and oregano and cook for about 5 minutes, until soft. Add the stock, vinegar, lentils and passata. Stir to combine, then reduce the heat to medium-low. Simmer uncovered for 25 minutes, stirring every 5 minutes or so.

3. While the sauce cooks, place the potatoes and garlic into another large saucepan. Cover with water and bring to the boil over high heat. Reduce the heat slightly and cook for 15–20 minutes, until the potatoes are very soft. Drain well and return to the saucepan. Add the olive oil and mash until smooth.

4. Remove the roasted vegetables from the oven and reduce the oven temperature to 160°C (fan-forced). Remove the lentil sauce from the heat, then tip the vegetables into the sauce and season with pepper if desired. Stir everything together.

5. Tip the lentil mixture into a large baking dish (30 cm × 20 cm, approx.). Spread the garlic mashed potato evenly over the top and use a fork to create ridges in the surface, to help it crisp up in the oven.

6. Bake for 30 minutes, until the mash is lightly golden on top. Cool slightly before serving.

LOADED SWEET POTATOES (with video)

A quick and easy winter warmer! Feel free to substitute the filling ingredients with whatever you have on hand or in the pantry. This recipe makes a satisfying meal for two, or if your sweet potatoes are larger this can be shared between four as a side. Omit the yoghurt if you would like to make this a vegan meal.

Serves 2–4

Prep Time: 10 minutes
Cooking Time: 10 minutes

2 sweet potatoes, washed and dried
250 g cherry tomatoes, chopped
½ × 400 g tin corn kernels, drained
½ × 400 g tin black beans, rinsed and drained
½ × 400 g tin red kidney beans, rinsed and drained
1 clove garlic, crushed
Juice of 1 lime
1 tablespoon olive oil
Sprinkle of paprika
Sprinkle of ground cumin
Handful of flat-leaf parsley and/or coriander leaves, chopped
1 avocado, mashed, to serve
4 tablespoons Greek yoghurt, to serve

1. Use a small knife to stab holes into the top of each sweet potato. Place onto a large plate. Microwave on high for 8–10 minutes, until the flesh is soft and fragrant. Each microwave will vary, so check the potatoes every few minutes and turn over if necessary. Set aside to cool slightly.
2. Meanwhile, combine the tomatoes, corn, black beans, kidney beans, garlic, lime juice, oil, paprika and cumin in a mixing bowl. Season with salt and pepper if desired. Stir well to combine, then stir in the herbs.

3. Cut the sweet potatoes lengthways along the top, without cutting all the way through. Transfer to serving plates.

4. Fill each sweet potato with the bean mixture – make sure to load them up. Top with a dollop each of avocado and yoghurt to serve.

EASY PEASY PASTA (with video)

As the name suggests this is an easy pasta recipe that can be whipped up quickly with minimal ingredients. It is best eaten immediately after cooking. As an option, add a dash of finely grated lemon zest and some fresh parsley for an extra hit of flavour.

Serves 4

Prep Time: 5 minutes
Cooking Time: 10 minutes

400 g pasta (we used wholemeal spaghetti)
1½ cups (180 g) frozen peas, thawed
3 eggs
½ cup (100 g) smooth ricotta
½ cup (40 g) finely grated parmesan

1. Bring a large saucepan of water to the boil over high heat. Add the pasta and cook for 8–10 minutes, until al dente (still slightly firm to the bite).
2. Reserve 1 cup (250 ml) of the pasta water and set aside. Stir the peas into the pasta and stand for 1 minute. Drain well, then return the pasta and peas to the saucepan.
3. While the pasta is cooking, crack the eggs into a mixing bowl. Add the ricotta and parmesan, and season with freshly ground black pepper if desired. Whisk well to combine.
4. Add the whisked egg mixture to the saucepan, along with half the reserved pasta water. Working quickly, use tongs to combine the pasta and the sauce. The pasta and peas should still be hot which will ensure that the eggs cook through.
5. Stir in some extra pasta water if desired, to create a thinner sauce consistency. Once everything is combined and the sauce evenly coats the pasta, divide between bowls and serve immediately.

BAKED LEMON CHICKEN (with video)

A winning chicken dinner! This is super simple to prepare, and baking everything together in one dish means less washing up! Serve with a simple side of greens such as grilled broccolini, asparagus or green beans. Alternatively, serve with a substantial salad and some brown rice, and this will feed a crowd.

Serves 6

Prep Time: 5 minutes
Cooking Time: 30 minutes

4 large chicken breast fillets
2 lemons, quartered
200 g haloumi, thickly sliced
2 tablespoons olive oil
2 tablespoons honey
Generous sprinkle of dried oregano

1. Preheat the oven to 200°C (fan-forced). Line a large baking dish with baking paper.
2. Arrange the chicken in the dish. Add the lemon quarters and the haloumi slices. Drizzle with the olive oil and honey, and add a generous sprinkle of oregano.
3. Bake for 25–30 minutes, until the chicken is cooked through and the haloumi is golden. If the haloumi or lemon are getting too golden or burnt, you can cover the dish with foil and return to the oven for the remaining cooking time.
4. Squeeze the roasted lemon quarters over the chicken and season with freshly ground black pepper if desired. Cut the chicken into slices to serve.

RICH TOMATO STEW WITH HALOUMI (with video)

A hearty and flavoursome meal – this recipe is easier to prepare than it sounds and works well for a mid-week dinner. Why not double the quantities so that you can portion out leftovers and freeze, ready to reheat for weekday lunches?

Serves 4

Prep Time: 15 minutes
Cooking Time: 30 minutes

1 cup (200 g) brown rice
¼ cup (60 ml) olive oil
1 red onion, finely chopped
2 cloves garlic, minced
1 small eggplant, chopped
2 tablespoons tomato paste
250 g cherry tomatoes, halved
1 teaspoon ground cinnamon
2 tablespoons red wine vinegar
400 g tin cherry tomatoes
250 g haloumi, cut into small cubes
400 g tin brown lentils, rinsed and drained

1. Cook the rice in a large saucepan of boiling water for 30 minutes, until tender. Drain well.
2. Meanwhile, heat the olive oil in a large saucepan over medium heat. Add the onion and garlic. Cook, stirring occasionally, for 5 minutes or until soft and lightly golden. Add the eggplant and cook for a further 5 minutes, stirring occasionally.

3. Add the tomato paste, fresh cherry tomatoes, cinnamon, vinegar and the tinned cherry tomatoes. Stir well to combine. Increase the heat to high, and cook for 5–10 minutes, stirring occasionally until the sauce is thickened. Add the haloumi and cook for a further 5 minutes, until heated through.

4. Sir the lentils through the brown rice. Divide between serving bowls. Spoon the haloumi mixture over and serve immediately.

CHICKPEA PASTA (with video)

This is a great weeknight dinner when there's nothing in the fridge and everyone is starving. Almost all the ingredients are pantry staples!

Serves 4

Prep Time: 10 minutes
Cooking Time: 25 minutes

2 tablespoons olive oil
3 cloves garlic, finely chopped
¼ cup (70 g) tomato paste
½ × 400 g tin chickpeas, rinsed and drained
400 g small wholemeal pasta (any variety is fine – allow your child to choose)
3 cups (750 ml) salt-reduced stock (any type) or water
1 small red chilli, finely chopped (see Note)
1 sprig rosemary, leaves stripped (see Note)

1. Heat the olive oil in a deep frying pan or large saucepan over medium heat. Add the garlic and cook, stirring, for about 30 seconds or until lightly golden. Add the tomato paste, then cook, stirring, for 2 minutes. Add the chickpeas and cook for a further 5 minutes.
2. Add the pasta and pour in the stock or water. Bring to the boil and cook for about 12 minutes, until the pasta is al dente (still slightly firm to the bite). If you think the pan is drying out, add another ½ cup (125 ml) water to ensure the pasta cooks.
3. It's ready to eat now if you like a soupy consistency, or cook a little longer until the liquid has reduced to more like a sauce. Stir in the chilli and rosemary and serve.

Note: Use a generous shake of dried chilli flakes and dried rosemary instead of the fresh option, if that is what you have on hand.

CHICKPEA HARISSA BAKE (with video)

A one-pot vegetable wonder! Harissa is a hot chilli paste that adds heat and lots of flavour to a dish, so it's important to sample the heat or modify the quantity before serving to young children. This recipe results in a hearty and delicious vegan meal and is super simple to put together. It stores well in the fridge so can be prepared in advance. You could also serve this as a side dish with roast meat and some couscous.

Serves 4 (or 8 as a side)

Prep Time: 10 minutes
Cooking Time: 40 minutes

2 carrots, chopped
1 eggplant, chopped
1 sweet potato, chopped
4 cloves garlic, peeled
2 × 400 g tins chickpeas, rinsed and drained
¼ cup (60 ml) olive oil
1 teaspoon ground cumin
1 teaspoon ground cinnamon
1 tablespoon harissa paste
Flat-leaf parsley leaves, chopped, to serve

1. Preheat the oven to 190°C (fan-forced).
2. Place the carrot, eggplant, sweet potato, garlic and chickpeas into a large baking dish (30 cm × 20 cm, approx.). Drizzle with the oil and sprinkle over the cumin and cinnamon. Add the harissa paste and season with pepper if desired.
3. Stir all the ingredients well to combine and coat everything with the harissa and spices. You can use your hands if you like.
4. Bake for 35–40 minutes, giving everything a good stir halfway through, until the vegetables are golden on the edges and the sweet potato is soft. Top with parsley to serve.

BEEF AND LENTIL BOLOGNAISE

A staple pasta recipe to have in your repertoire. The addition of lentils means you use less meat in this recipe, but you won't even notice the difference. Feel free to also bulk up the pasta sauce by adding even more veggies, such as mushrooms.

Serves 4

Prep Time: 15 minutes
Cooking Time: 30 minutes

300 g wholemeal spiral pasta
1 tablespoon olive oil
1 clove garlic, crushed
1 brown onion, finely diced
1 carrot, finely diced
1 teaspoon ground cumin
1 teaspoon dried oregano
250 g lean beef mince
1 tablespoon tomato paste
400 g tin crushed tomatoes
½ cup (125 ml) vegetable stock
400 g tin brown lentils, rinsed and drained
Handful of basil leaves, to serve

1. Bring a large saucepan of water to the boil over high heat. Add the pasta and cook for about 12 minutes, until al dente (still slightly firm to the bite). Drain.
2. Meanwhile, heat the olive oil in a large saucepan over medium heat. Add the garlic and onion and cook for 5 minutes or until soft. Add the carrot, cumin and oregano and cook for another 5 minutes, stirring occasionally.

3. Add the mince and cook, breaking up any lumps with a wooden spoon, until browned. Stir in the tomato paste and cook for 1 minute, then stir in the tomatoes and stock. Bring to a simmer and cook for 10–15 minutes, until thickened.

4. Stir in the lentils and season with freshly ground black pepper if desired. Cook for a couple more minutes, until the lentils have heated through.

5. Divide the pasta between 4 serving bowls and top with the bolognaise sauce. Sprinkle with torn basil leaves and serve.

SAN CHOY BOW

These delicious lettuce wraps contain lots of veggies in a delicious savoury mince sauce. This recipe is also a perfect weeknight dinner idea as it requires minimal cooking time.

Serves 4

Prep Time: 15 minutes
Cooking Time: 15 minutes

8 large iceberg lettuce leaves (or 12–16 small leaves)
1 tablespoon canola oil
1 small brown onion, diced
1 teaspoon finely grated ginger
2 cloves garlic, crushed
1 carrot, diced
1 red capsicum, diced
350 g lean beef mince
1 cup (100 g) button mushrooms, chopped
5 baby corn spears, chopped
3 spring onions, sliced
2 tablespoons gluten-free soy sauce (or tamari)
2 tablespoons gluten-free oyster sauce
1 teaspoon sesame oil
1 cup (80 g) beansprouts
1 tablespoon sesame seeds
1 tablespoon unsalted roasted peanuts, chopped

1. Wash and dry the iceberg lettuce leaves and store in the fridge so that they are chilled before serving.
2. Heat the canola oil in a large frying pan over high heat. Add the onion and cook for 2 minutes. Add the ginger, garlic, carrot and capsicum and continue to cook for another 3 minutes, stirring often. Add the mince and cook, breaking up any lumps with a wooden spoon, until browned. Stir in the mushrooms, baby corn and spring onions and cook for another 5 minutes.

3. Combine the soy sauce, oyster sauce and sesame oil in a small bowl. Pour over the mince mixture and stir to combine. Remove from the heat.

4. Divide the mixture evenly between the lettuce leaves and top with the beansprouts, sesame seeds and peanuts. Alternatively, spoon the mince mixture into a large bowl and have the lettuce leaves and toppings on the dining table so diners can serve themselves.

HEALTHY NACHOS

This version is made with beef mince, but you can easily make it vegetarian by replacing the beef with another tin of red kidney beans.

Serves 8

Prep Time: 15 minutes
Cooking Time: 25 minutes

1 tablespoon olive oil
1 brown onion, finely chopped
500 g lean beef mince
400 g tin red kidney beans, rinsed and drained
1 red chilli, finely chopped
2 tablespoons tomato paste
2 × 400 g tins crushed tomatoes with Italian herbs (or plain if you prefer)
230 g packet wholegrain tortilla or corn chips
⅓ cup (40 g) grated cheddar cheese
1 avocado, diced
Handful of coriander leaves (see Note)

1. Preheat the oven to 180°C (fan-forced).
2. Heat the olive oil in a large frying pan over medium heat, add the onion and cook for 3 minutes or until softened.
3. Add the mince and cook, breaking up any lumps with a wooden spoon, until browned.
4. Stir in the kidney beans, chilli, tomato paste and tomatoes. Reduce the heat to low and simmer for 10 minutes or until the mixture thickens.
5. Spread the tortilla chips across two deep baking trays. Top with the mince mixture and sprinkle over the grated cheese.
6. Bake for about 8 minutes or until the cheese is melted.
7. Serve topped with the avocado and coriander.

Note: If you prefer your nachos crunchy, sprinkle some corn chips on top of the mince sauce as well. You can also replace the coriander with flat-leaf parsley leaves, baby rocket or torn kale.

GARLIC PRAWNS WITH ZUCCHINI NOODLES

Prawns are a terrific protein source, and are super satisfying cooked in this garlic sauce. This recipe is also great to use up some stale bread for the breadcrumbs – or omit them altogether for a gluten-free version of this meal. If you are short on time, supermarkets are now stocking zucchini noodles in the fresh or frozen sections which you can substitute in this recipe.

Serves 4

Prep Time: 10 minutes
Cooking Time: 10 minutes

2–3 slices stale wholegrain or sourdough bread, toasted
3 tablespoons olive oil
1 tablespoon dried oregano
Handful of basil leaves, plus extra to serve
3 cloves garlic, crushed
Sprinkle of dried chilli flakes
250 g cherry tomatoes, halved
350 g uncooked peeled prawns, deveined, without tails
2 zucchini, spiralised

1. Break the toasted bread into a blender and pulse into coarse breadcrumbs. Alternatively, you can crumble into breadcrumbs with your hands.
2. Heat 1 tablespoon of the olive oil in a large non-stick frying pan over high heat. Add the breadcrumbs and cook for 5 minutes, stirring often, until golden. Sprinkle in the oregano and tear in the basil leaves. Remove the breadcrumb mixture from the pan, set aside, and give the pan a quick wipe.
3. Heat the remaining oil in the pan over medium heat. Add the garlic and chilli flakes. Cook for 1 minute, until fragrant, then add the cherry tomatoes. Increase the heat to high and add the prawns. Cook for 3–4 minutes, turning occasionally, until the prawns change colour and are cooked through. Remove from the heat.

4. Add the zucchini to the pan and stir through. The residual heat in the pan will soften the zucchini noodles. Season with freshly ground black pepper if desired.

5. Divide the prawn and zucchini noodles between 4 serving bowls. Sprinkle the breadcrumb mixture over the top and scatter with the extra basil leaves. Serve immediately.

FISH TACOS

Why not enjoy Taco Tuesday at home this week? These fish tacos are easy to prepare and are perfect if you are feeding a crowd – just cook the fish and prepare the veggies, then serve everything on the table for everyone to assemble their own dinner.

Serves 4

Prep Time: 10 minutes
Cooking Time: 10 minutes

3 skinless, boneless salmon fillets
1 tablespoon red curry paste
8 mini wholemeal tortillas
1 large Lebanese cucumber, peeled into thin ribbons
1 bag (60 g) mixed lettuce leaves
1 lemon, quartered, to serve

Minted yoghurt
5 tablespoons Greek yoghurt
¼ Lebanese cucumber, finely diced
Handful of mint leaves, chopped
Juice of ½ lemon

1. Heat a large non-stick frying pan over medium heat. Fry the salmon fillets for 3–4 minutes, then turn over and cook on the other side for 4–5 minutes. (This will require longer if you prefer your fish cooked through.) While the salmon is cooking use a pastry brush to spread the red curry paste over all sides of the fillets.
2. Meanwhile, to prepare the minted yoghurt, combine all the ingredients in a small bowl and stir to combine.
3. Transfer the salmon to a large plate and use a fork to flake into large chunks.
4. Serve the fish with the tortillas, cucumber strips, mixed lettuce leaves and the minted yoghurt. Diners can assemble into tacos and top with a squeeze of lemon.

EASY WHOLEMEAL PASTA WITH TURKEY MINCE

A simple and healthy meal that is perfect to put together for a weeknight dinner when you are short on time. Turkey mince is a great lean protein source, so why not give it a try to add some variety into your diet. This meal also works well to make in advance, and portion into containers to freeze for lunches or dinners later in the week.

Serves 4

Prep Time: 10 minutes
Cooking Time: 15 minutes

300 g wholemeal penne
300 g green beans, trimmed and halved
1 tablespoon olive oil
1 red onion, finely diced
2 cloves garlic, crushed
300 g lean turkey breast mince
250 g cherry tomatoes, halved
Sprinkle of dried chilli flakes (add extra for more of a flavour kick)
2 tablespoons red wine vinegar
1 bag (60 g) baby spinach leaves
Cottage cheese, to serve

1. Bring a large saucepan of water to the boil over high heat. Add the penne and cook for about 12 minutes, until al dente (still slightly firm to the bite). Remove from the heat, then add the green beans. Stand for a couple of minutes then drain and transfer to a large bowl.
2. Meanwhile, heat the olive oil in a non-stick frying pan over medium heat. Add the onion and garlic and cook for 5 minutes, until softened. Add the turkey mince and cook, breaking up any lumps with a wooden spoon, until browned. Stir in the tomatoes, chilli flakes and red wine vinegar.

3. Simmer the mixture for 5 minutes. Use a spoon to crush the tomatoes so they are softened and create a sauce.

4. Add the turkey mince mixture to the pasta and beans. Add the baby spinach and stir to combine. Divide between 4 serving bowls then top with the cottage cheese and some freshly ground black pepper if desired.

SNACKS AND SWEET TREATS

APPLE SLICE 'DONUTS'

A great after school snack for the whole family. For a nut-free option, you can swap the peanut butter for yoghurt. Get creative with the donut toppings – we used granola, sunflower seeds and dark chocolate chips.

Makes 10

Prep Time: 10 minutes

2 large pink lady apples
3 tablespoons natural 100% peanut butter
3 tablespoons of assorted toppings

1. Use an apple corer to remove the core of each apple.
2. Place the apple on its side so that the empty core is parallel to your chopping board. Trim both ends of the apple, then slice the apple into 5 even slices.
3. Place the apple slices – cut side facing up – onto a flat chopping board or plate.
4. Spread the top of each slice with peanut butter.
5. Sprinkle the assorted toppings on top of the peanut butter, and serve the apple 'donuts' immediately.

SPINACH LOAF

This hearty and nourishing green loaf is delicious enjoyed on its own as a snack, or as a substitute for your regular loaf of bread. Why not try it topped with smashed avocado, fried eggs and some dried chilli flakes, or toasted and served alongside some homemade baked beans. Delicious!

Serves 8

Prep Time: 10 minutes
Cooking Time: 45 minutes

120–150 g baby spinach or chopped silverbeet leaves
3 eggs
⅔ cup (160 ml) milk
¼ cup (60 ml) olive oil
2 cups (320 g) wholemeal self-raising flour
Pinch of ground cumin
Pinch of paprika
½ cup (50 g) grated mozzarella

1. Preheat the oven to 180°C (fan-forced). Lightly grease a loaf tin (24 cm × 14 cm, approx.) and line with baking paper, extending over the two long sides.
2. Place the spinach or silverbeet, eggs, milk and olive oil into a large blender. Using the pulse button, blend the mixture in short bursts until the ingredients are combined into a lumpy green mixture. Pour into a large mixing bowl.
3. Gently fold in the flour, cumin, paprika and mozzarella. Try to mix until only just combined, as overmixing will result in a tough-textured loaf. Pour into the prepared tin.
4. Bake for 40–45 minutes, until the loaf has risen and springs back to the touch. If you aren't sure, insert a skewer into the centre of the loaf – it should come out clean to indicate that it is cooked through.
5. Cool completely in the tin, then use the paper to lift it out. Cut into thick slices to serve. Store in an airtight container in the fridge for up to 5 days.

GF DF BANANA LOAF

This is a gluten-free and dairy-free recipe that results in a delicious banana loaf.

Serves 8

Prep Time: 10 minutes
Cooking Time: 45 minutes

3 overripe bananas
2 eggs
½ cup (125 ml) soy milk
2 tablespoons olive oil
1 tablespoon honey
2 cups (240 g) ground almonds
½ cup (70 g) ground flaxseed
2 teaspoons ground cinnamon
1½ teaspoons baking powder
¼ cup (25 g) walnuts, toasted and roughly chopped

1. Preheat the oven to 160°C (fan-forced). Lightly grease a loaf tin (24 cm × 14 cm, approx.) and line with baking paper, extending over the two long sides.
2. Place the bananas into a large mixing bowl and mash well with a fork. Add the eggs, soy milk, olive oil and honey. Mix well to combine.
3. Add the ground almonds and flaxseed, cinnamon, baking powder and walnuts. Fold all ingredients together until well combined. Pour the batter into the prepared tin.
4. Bake for 40–45 minutes, until risen, golden and springy to a gentle touch in the centre. Cool slightly in the tin.
5. Transfer to a wire rack to cool completely. Cut into thick slices to serve. Store leftover loaf in an airtight container for up to 3 days at room temperature.

BANANA OAT BARS

These bars are a delicious healthy snack, perfect for both adults and children.

Makes 15

Prep Time: 10 minutes
Cooking Time: 30 minutes

2 overripe bananas
1 egg
⅓ cup (80 ml) olive oil
2 tablespoons honey, plus extra to serve (optional)
1 heaped tablespoon 100% natural peanut or almond butter
1 cup (90 g) rolled oats
½ cup (80 g) wholemeal self-raising flour
1 tablespoon pepitas, plus extra to serve (optional)
1 tablespoon sunflower seeds, plus extra to serve (optional)
2 tablespoons goji berries, or other dried fruit

1. Preheat the oven to 180°C (fan-forced). Lightly grease a 20 cm square cake tin and line with baking paper, extending over 2 sides.
2. Place the bananas into a large mixing bowl and mash well with a fork. Add the egg and mix into the banana. Add the olive oil, honey and peanut butter and mix well to combine.
3. Gently fold in the oats, flour, pepitas, sunflower seeds and goji berries. Pour the batter into the prepared tin.
4. Bake for 30 minutes, until golden and firm to the touch. Set aside to cool completely in the tin.
5. Lift out and slice into 15 bars. If you like, drizzle with honey and sprinkle with extra pepitas and sunflower seeds before serving. Store in an airtight container in the fridge for up to 1 week.

ZUCCHINI AND CORN SLICE

This is a quick recipe to whip up, and it is a great slice for kids to enjoy as a snack or as part of their school lunchbox.

Makes 15

Prep Time: 10 minutes
Cooking Time: 40 minutes

6 eggs
1 cup (250 ml) milk
1 cup (160 g) wholemeal self-raising flour
2 large zucchini, grated
1 cup (160 g) frozen corn kernels
Handful of fresh herb leaves, such as coriander or mint
½ cup (60 g) grated cheddar cheese (optional)

1. Preheat the oven to 180°C (fan-forced). Lightly grease a 26 cm × 16 cm (base) slice tin and line with baking paper, extending over the two long sides.
2. Whisk the eggs and milk together in a large mixing bowl. Add the flour and whisk just until smooth. Add the zucchini, corn, herbs and cheese, if using. Stir well to combine. Pour the batter into the prepared tin.
3. Bake for 35–40 minutes, until puffed up and golden. Set aside to cool completely in the tin.
4. Lift out and cut into squares to serve. Store in an airtight container in the fridge for up to 3 days.

BERRY FROZEN YOGHURT DROPS

A delicious snack to prepare in advance and keep in the freezer until needed. These are perfect for your little ones to enjoy as the weather gets hotter. This recipe uses berries, but you could also substitute other seasonal fruit of your choice.

Makes about 30

Prep Time: 10 minutes + 2 hours freezing

½ cup (75 g) mixed berries (see Note)
1 cup (280 g) Greek yoghurt

1. Lightly grease 2 baking trays and line with baking paper. Combine the berries and yoghurt in a small blender. Blend until smooth.
2. Use a teaspoon to dollop spoonfuls of the yoghurt mixture onto the baking trays. Continue until all the yoghurt mixture has been used.
3. Carefully transfer the trays to the freezer, ensuring that they are level. Freeze for about 2 hours, until firm.
4. Remove the yoghurt drops from the trays and place into an airtight container, then return to the freezer. Take out and serve frozen as needed.

Note: Use a mixture of strawberries, blueberries and raspberries, or just one type if you prefer. You can also use frozen berries, just let them thaw slightly before blending.

BABY BANANA MUFFINS

These muffins are great to make for young children. They are miniature size, making them perfect for little fingers to grab them. You can freeze them and they will thaw fairly quickly, so pop one in their lunchbox or bag for a day out and you won't have to resort to buying snacks.

Makes 24

Prep Time: 10 minutes
Cooking Time: 15 minutes

Olive oil spray
½ cup (125 ml) milk
Juice of ½ lemon
2 large overripe bananas
2 eggs
¼ cup (70 g) Greek yoghurt
⅓ cup (80 ml) olive oil
1¾ cups (280 g) wholemeal self-raising flour
Pinch of ground cinnamon

1. Preheat the oven to 160°C (fan-forced). Lightly grease two 12-hole mini muffin trays with olive oil spray. Combine the milk and lemon juice in a jug and set aside for a few minutes.
2. Place the bananas into a large mixing bowl and mash well with a fork. Add the eggs and mix into the banana until well combined. Add the yoghurt and olive oil, then pour in the milk mixture. Mix until well combined.
3. Add the flour and cinnamon, then fold together gently until just combined (not overmixing the batter will result in light, tender muffins). Spoon the batter evenly into the prepared trays.

4. Bake for 15 minutes, until risen, golden and springy to a gentle touch. Set aside to cool in the trays for 5 minutes.

5. Transfer the muffins to a wire rack to cool completely. Store in an airtight container for up to 2 days, or wrap individually in foil and freeze in an airtight freezer bag for up to 3 weeks.

Note: Adding lemon juice to the milk makes it curdle slightly and it ends up being like buttermilk. This will make the muffins really tender.

KID-FRIENDLY BANANA PINWHEELS

This is a quick and easy snack that you can whip up for your kids, and for you too!

Makes 8–10

Prep Time: 5 minutes

1 wholegrain wrap or tortilla
1 heaped tablespoon 100% natural peanut butter
1 large banana

1. Lay out the wrap on a flat surface. Spread evenly with the peanut butter.
2. Place the banana along the left side of the wrap. Fold the left edge over the banana. Roll towards the right to enclose the whole banana, ensuring that you wrap the banana tightly. Press the edge of the wrap down firmly at the end to secure it.
3. Use a sharp knife to slice the wrapped banana into thick pinwheels. Place onto the plate with the cut side facing up. Serve immediately.

SPINACH MUFFINS

A delicious savoury muffin recipe, perfect for a lunchbox snack. The spinach is chopped up and has a mild flavour, so your kids will also enjoy these muffins. If you want to make this recipe for your little ones, you could also bake this mixture in mini muffin trays and cook for 10–12 minutes.

Makes 16

Prep Time: 10 minutes
Cooking Time: 20 minutes

Olive oil spray
150–200 g baby spinach leaves
2 eggs
¾ cup (210 g) Greek yoghurt
½ cup (125 ml) milk
½ cup (55 g) grated cheddar cheese or mozzarella
2 cups (320 g) wholemeal self-raising flour

1. Preheat the oven to 180°C (fan-forced). Lightly grease 16 holes of two 12-hole medium muffin trays with olive oil spray.
2. Place the baby spinach into a large mixing bowl and use scissors to roughly chop it into small pieces.
3. Add the eggs and mix well to combine. Stir in the yoghurt, milk and cheese.
4. Gently mix in the flour. Try to mix until only just combined, as overmixing will result in a tough-textured muffin.
5. Divide the muffin mixture between the 16 greased holes.
6. Bake for 20 minutes, until the muffins have risen, are lightly golden and springy to the touch. Set aside to cool in the trays for 5 minutes.
7. Transfer the muffins to a wire rack to cool completely. Store leftover muffins in an airtight container for up to 2 days or wrap individually in foil and freeze in an airtight freezer bag for up to 3 weeks.

MINI BANANA MUFFINS

These muffins taste like little sweet frittatas, perfect as a healthy snack. We used colourful mini patty pans to make these appealing for little kids, but they are optional. If you are making these for your baby make sure you peel off the patty pan before serving.

Makes 24

Prep Time: 10 minutes
Cooking Time: 15 minutes

1 cup (150 g) mixed berries (raspberries, blueberries, chopped strawberries)
2 overripe bananas
4 eggs
Mini patty pans (optional)

1. Preheat the oven to 180°C (fan-forced). Line two 12-hole mini muffin trays with patty pans (or lightly grease with olive oil spray).
2. Divide the berries between patty pans. Place the bananas into a mixing bowl and use a fork to mash until smooth (it is okay if a few small lumps remain).
3. Add the eggs and mix until well combined. Pour the egg mixture into each patty pan.
4. Bake for 15 minutes. The muffins will rise up and then sink again once removed from the oven. Cool completely before serving. Store leftover muffins in an airtight container for up to 2 days, or wrap individually in foil and freeze in an airtight freezer bag for up to 3 weeks.

TOMATO, FETA AND PINE NUT MUFFINS

A delicious savoury muffin recipe, perfect to be enjoyed by the whole family. These muffins are best served fresh but they can also be frozen in order to enjoy later.

Makes 12

Prep Time: 15 minutes
Cooking Time: 40 minutes

Olive oil spray
200 g grape tomatoes, halved
1 egg
1 cup (250 ml) milk
¼ cup (60 g) sour cream
¼ cup (60 ml) olive oil
2 tablespoons Homemade Basil Pesto (page 200)
50 g feta, crumbled
¼ cup (40 g) pine nuts, toasted
2 cups (320 g) wholemeal self-raising flour

1. Preheat the oven to 170°C (fan-forced). Lightly grease a 12-hole medium muffin tray with olive oil spray. Line a baking tray with baking paper.
2. Place the tomato halves onto the prepared baking tray and roast for 10–15 minutes, until softened. Set aside to cool slightly.
3. In a large mixing bowl whisk the egg, milk, sour cream and olive oil together until combined. Stir in the basil pesto. Mix in the roasted tomatoes, the feta and half the pine nuts.
4. Gently fold in the flour until just combined. Try to stir as few times as possible, as handling gently will result in light and fluffy muffins.
5. Divide the muffin mixture evenly between the holes in the tray. Top with the remaining pine nuts.

6. Bake for 25 minutes or until the muffins are risen, golden and springy to a gentle touch.

7. Set aside to cool slightly before removing the muffins from the tray. Store leftover muffins in an airtight container for up to 2 days or wrap individually in foil and freeze in an airtight freezer bag for up to 3 weeks.

ENERGY BALLS

These energy balls are a delicious and filling snack for when you are on the go.

Makes about 40

Prep Time: 15 minutes

2½ cups (225 g) rolled oats
1 cup (120 g) ground almonds
400 g jar 100% natural peanut butter (smooth)
300 g honey
¼ cup (20 g) desiccated coconut

1. Place the oats into a blender and use the pulse button to blend in short bursts until the oats resemble the consistency of flour.
2. Pour the oat flour into a large mixing bowl. Add the ground almonds, peanut butter and honey. Mix everything well to combine and ensure there are no lumps.
3. Place the coconut into a small bowl. Take a level tablespoon of mixture and roll into a ball. Roll the ball in the desiccated coconut to coat. Tap off excess coconut, then place ball onto a large flat tray. Repeat with remaining mixture and coconut.
4. Store in an airtight container in the fridge for up to one week, or in the freezer for a month.

Tip: Have all ingredients at room temperature before making this recipe, as it will ensure you can combine them easily.

RASPBERRY CRUMBLE SLICE

A yummy slice that both children and adults will enjoy when packed as a lunchbox snack! Raspberries and blueberries work best but feel free to substitute whatever frozen berries you can find.

Makes 15

Prep Time: 15 minutes
Cooking Time: 35 minutes

500 g frozen raspberries (or mixed berries)
2 tablespoons chia seeds
3 tablespoons honey
1½ cups (180 g) ground almonds
¾ cup (120 g) wholemeal plain flour
1 cup (90 g) rolled oats
⅓ cup (80 ml) olive oil

1. Preheat the oven to 180°C (fan-forced). Lightly grease a 26 cm × 16 cm (base) slice tin and line with baking paper, extending over the two long sides.
2. Place the frozen berries into a saucepan over medium-low heat. Add the chia seeds and 1 tablespoon of the honey. Heat for 5–10 minutes, until completely thawed and the mixture is thick. Some berries should remain whole, and the rest will become pulpy. Remove from the heat and set aside.
3. Meanwhile, place the ground almonds, flour and oats into a mixing bowl. Add the olive oil and remaining 2 tablespoons of honey. Stir well to combine.
4. The mixture should be crumbly but come together when pinched. Spread two-thirds of the crumble mixture into the prepared tin and use the back of a spoon to press to form the base of the slice.
5. Bake the base for 10 minutes or until lightly golden. Remove from the oven and top with the berry mixture. Sprinkle with the remaining crumble mixture.

6. Bake for a further 25 minutes, until the berries are bubbling up through the topping and it is golden.

7. Set aside to cool completely in the tin. Cut into squares to serve. Store in an airtight container in the fridge for up to 5 days, or freeze in an airtight freezer bag for up to 3 weeks.

STRAWBERRY BANANA MUFFINS

These muffins make a great morning or afternoon snack and are convenient to pack with you on the go or for a snack at work. The bananas and strawberries make them super moist and provide just the right amount of fruity flavour and sweetness.

Makes 12

Prep Time: 10 minutes
Cooking Time: 20 minutes

Olive oil spray
3 overripe bananas
½ cup (140 g) Greek yoghurt
1 tablespoon honey
2 eggs
½ cup (about 100 g) strawberries, chopped into small pieces
1¾ cup (280 g) wholemeal self-raising flour
1 teaspoon baking powder
1 teaspoon ground cinnamon

1. Preheat the oven to 180°C (fan-forced). Lightly grease a 12-hole medium muffin tray with olive oil spray.
2. Mash the bananas in a large bowl. Add the yoghurt, honey and eggs and mix well. Stir in the chopped strawberries.
3. Add the flour, baking powder and cinnamon and fold through gently to combine. Ensure there are no lumps of flour but be careful not to overmix as this will result in tough muffins. Spoon the mixture into the prepared tray.
4. Bake for 20 minutes, until risen, lightly golden and springy to a gentle touch. Set aside to cool in the tray for 5 minutes.
5. Transfer the muffins to a wire rack to cool completely. Store in an airtight container in the fridge for up to 5 days, or wrap individually in foil and freeze in an airtight freezer bag for up to 3 weeks.

Note: Make 24 mini muffins if you prefer, and bake for 10–12 minutes. These can be made gluten-free by substituting a gluten-free flour.

PEAR MUFFINS (with video)

Do you have some sad old overripe pears lying around? This recipe is the perfect way to use them up! Once pears are a bit bruised or soft you can store them in the fridge until you are ready to make this recipe. This recipe uses half rolled oats and half wholemeal flour which gives the muffins a lovely texture.

Makes 12

Prep Time: 15 minutes
Cooking Time: 15 minutes

Olive oil spray
1 cup (90 g) rolled oats
¾ cup (180 ml) milk
¼ cup (60 ml) olive oil
½ cup (180 g) honey
1 egg
1 teaspoon vanilla extract
2 large or 4 small overripe pears, cored and chopped
1 cup (160 g) wholemeal plain flour
1 teaspoon baking powder
½ teaspoon bicarb soda
1 teaspoon ground cinnamon
Pinch of salt

1. Preheat the oven to 190°C (fan-forced). Lightly grease a 12-hole medium muffin tray with olive oil spray.
2. Combine the oats, milk and ¼ cup (60 ml) water in a jug. Stir to combine, then set aside to sit for 5–10 minutes so the oats can soak up the liquid.
3. Place the oil, honey, egg, vanilla and soaked oat mixture into a large mixing bowl. Stir well to combine. Add the chopped pears, flour, baking powder, bicarb soda, cinnamon and salt.

4. Use a spatula to gently fold all the ingredients together. Ensure everything is combined but be careful not to overmix as this will result in tough-textured muffins. Spoon batter evenly into the prepared tray.

5. Bake for 15 minutes, until risen, golden and springy to a gentle touch. Cool in the tray for 5 minutes, then transfer to a wire rack to cool completely.

6. Store in an airtight container for up to 2 days, or wrap individually in foil and freeze in an airtight freezer bag for up to 3 weeks.

LEMON LOAF

This loaf is a perfect treat to share with family or friends for morning or afternoon tea on special occasions.

Serves 8

Prep Time: 10 minutes
Cooking Time: 45 minutes

1 cup (280 g) Greek yoghurt
3 eggs
½ cup (180 g) honey
½ cup (125 ml) olive oil
2 teaspoons finely grated lemon zest
Juice of 2 lemons
1½ cups (240 g) wholemeal self-raising flour
½ teaspoon salt

1. Preheat the oven to 180°C (fan-forced). Lightly grease a 24 cm × 14 cm loaf tin and line with baking paper, extending over the two long sides.
2. Whisk the yoghurt, eggs, honey, olive oil, lemon zest and juice in a mixing bowl.
3. In another mixing bowl, combine the flour and salt. Make a well in the centre and pour in the wet ingredients. Use a whisk to slowly incorporate everything together, ensuring there are no lumps. Pour into the prepared tin.
4. Bake for about 45 minutes, until risen, lightly golden and cooked through (check the cake is cooked by inserting a wooden skewer into the middle, if it comes out clean then the cake is cooked). Cool slightly in the tin.
5. Transfer to a wire rack to cool completely, then cut into slices to serve. Store leftover loaf in an airtight container for up to 5 days.

BEAUTIFUL BANANA BREAD

This is a healthier version of a classic favourite. Most of the sweetness in this recipe comes from the bananas, with some honey added, so make sure that your bananas are overripe as they will be sweeter. This can also be sliced up and packaged as a portion-controlled snack to store in the freezer for when you need something sweet.

Serves 8

Prep Time: 10 minutes
Cooking Time: 50 minutes

3 overripe bananas, plus ½ a banana for the top (optional)
1 egg
⅓ cup (80 ml) olive oil
⅓ cup (120 g) honey
⅓ cup (80 ml) milk
1 teaspoon ground cinnamon
½ teaspoon ground nutmeg
1 teaspoon baking powder
1½ cups (240 g) wholemeal self-raising flour
¼ cup (25 g) chopped walnuts (optional)
Pinch of salt

1. Preheat the oven to 190°C (fan-forced). Lightly grease a 24 cm × 14 cm loaf tin and line with baking paper, extending over the two long sides.
2. Place the bananas into a large mixing bowl and mash well with a fork. Add the egg, olive oil, honey, milk, cinnamon, nutmeg and salt. Mix well to combine.
3. Add the baking powder, flour and walnuts, if using. Gently fold to combine the wet and dry ingredients together. Make sure there are no lumps remaining. Pour the batter into the prepared tin. If you like, lay half a banana cut-side-up on top of the batter.

4. Bake for 45–50 minutes, until golden on top and cooked through. You can test the loaf is cooked by inserting a skewer into the middle of the loaf, if it comes out clean then the loaf is ready. Cool slightly in the tin.

5. Transfer to a wire rack to cool for at least 15 minutes before slicing and serving. Store any leftover loaf in an airtight container for up to 5 days, or wrap slices individually in foil and freeze in an airtight freezer bag for up to 3 weeks.

APRICOT CHOC OAT BARS

These bars are a perfect on-the-go snack. Make up a batch and package them individually so that you know you are prepared when hunger strikes!

Makes 10

Prep Time: 15 minutes
Cooking Time: 25 minutes

¾ cup (105 g) pitted Medjool dates
½ cup (45 g) rolled oats
¼ cup (20 g) shredded coconut
1 teaspoon ground cinnamon
½ cup (70 g) pepitas
2 tablespoons chia seeds
5 dried apricots, chopped into small pieces
50 g dark chocolate (70%), chopped into small pieces

1. Preheat the oven to 170°C (fan-forced). Lightly grease a 26 cm × 16 cm (base) slice tin and line with baking paper, extending over the two long sides.
2. Place the dates and 1 cup (250 ml) water into a small saucepan over high heat and cook for about 5 minutes, until the dates soften and start to dissolve into the water. Turn off the heat and use a fork to mash the dates into a thick lumpy mixture. Set aside to cool until just warm.
3. Place all the remaining ingredients into a mixing bowl, then stir through the date mixture until everything is well combined. Press firmly into the prepared tin and smooth the surface.
4. Bake for 15–20 minutes, until set and browned on top. Set aside to cool completely in the tin.
5. Lift out and cut into 10 bars. Store in an airtight container for up to 5 days.

HOT CROSS BUN MUFFINS (with video)

Not quite hot cross buns – but muffins instead! They don't have the cross on top but they do have all the spicy, fruity flavours of a hot cross bun. These can be prepared in a flash and are perfect to share with family and friends at Easter (or anytime!). They are delicious served warm – either fresh from the oven or warmed up again before serving.

Makes 10

Prep Time: 10 minutes
Cooking Time: 15 minutes

1½ cups (240 g) wholemeal self-raising flour
1 teaspoon mixed spice
1 teaspoon ground cinnamon
1 teaspoon baking powder
½ cup (125 ml) milk
¼ cup (125 ml) olive oil
¼ cup (90 g) honey
1 egg
¾ cup (120 g) mixed dried fruit

1. Preheat the oven to 160°C (fan-forced). Lightly grease 10 holes of a 12-hole medium muffin tray.
2. Place the flour, spices and baking powder into a mixing bowl. Stir to combine. Use a fork to whisk the milk, olive oil, honey and egg in a jug.
3. Make a well in the centre of the dry ingredients, then pour in the wet ingredients. Add the dried fruit before mixing gently until just combined. Do not overmix as this will result in tough-textured muffins.
4. Divide the mixture evenly between the greased holes of the muffin tray.

5. Bake for 15 minutes, until golden brown and springy to a gentle touch. Cool in the tray for 5 minutes, then serve warm.
6. Store in an airtight container for up to 2 days, or wrap individually in foil and freeze in an airtight freezer bag for up to 3 weeks.

EGG AND VEGGIE MUFFINS (with video)

These frittata-style egg muffins are simple to make, and store well in the fridge or freezer. They are great to have as a snack, or you could serve a couple with a salad for lunch. You can add any vegetables or fresh herbs that you have on hand, just make sure to grate or chop the vegetables thinly to ensure they cook through.

Makes 12

Prep Time: 10 minutes
Cooking Time: 25 minutes

6 eggs
½ cup (125 ml) milk
¼ cup (30 g) ground almonds
½ large zucchini, grated
1 carrot, grated
¾ cup (90 g) frozen peas, thawed
½ cup (60 g) grated cheddar cheese

1. Preheat the oven to 180°C (fan-forced). Lightly grease a 12-hole medium muffin tray.
2. Crack the eggs into a large mixing bowl and add the milk and ground almonds. Whisk well to combine. Stir in the zucchini, carrot, peas and cheese.
3. Transfer the mixture from the bowl to a jug. Pour the mixture into the muffin holes, dividing evenly.
4. Bake for 20–25 minutes, until the muffins have risen, are lightly golden and springy to the touch. Set aside to cool in the trays for 5 minutes.
5. Serve warm, or transfer to a wire rack to cool completely. Store leftover muffins in an airtight container in the fridge for up to 2 days or wrap individually in foil and freeze in an airtight freezer bag for up to 3 weeks.

TAHINI NUT BARS (with video)

These bars make a great snack. Wrap in individual portions to have on hand when needed.

Makes 40

Prep Time: 10 minutes + 4 hours freezing
Cooking Time: 5 minutes

½ cup (140 g) tahini
½ cup (140 g) 100% natural peanut butter
⅓ cup (120 g) honey
1 cup (90 g) rolled oats
½ cup (75 g) sesame seeds
½ cup (80 g) dry roasted almonds, roughly chopped
1 teaspoon ground cinnamon

1. Place the tahini, peanut butter and honey into a small saucepan. Stir over low heat until melted and combined. Add 2 tablespoons of water to thin out the consistency slightly.
2. Mix the rolled oats, sesame seeds, almonds and cinnamon together in a mixing bowl. Make a well in the centre, add the tahini mixture and stir to combine
3. Lightly grease a 26 cm × 16 cm (base) slice tin and line with baking paper, extending over the two long sides. Spread the mixture evenly into the tin and use the back of a spoon to press the mixture down firmly.
4. Place the tin into the freezer for at least 4 hours to set. Lift from the tray and use a sharp knife to cut into small squares or bars.

Note: These can be stored in the fridge or freezer for a couple of weeks.

APPLE CRUMBLE

A delicious, filling and healthy dessert for those times when you feel like a sweet treat after dinner. This recipe is great for a large family, or you can divide all ingredients by six if you would like to make a dessert for one. You could also add some frozen berries or sliced stone fruit to the cooked apple mixture. It is a great dish to use up any overripe fruit you have.

Serves 6

Prep Time: 10 minutes
Cooking Time: 30 minutes

6 apples (see Note)
1 teaspoon ground cinnamon
1 teaspoon ground nutmeg
Finely grated zest of 1 orange
1 cup (90 g) rolled oats
½ cup (40 g) desiccated coconut
¼ cup (60 ml) olive oil
¼ cup (40 g) raw almonds, roughly chopped
Greek yoghurt, to serve

1. Preheat the oven to 180°C (fan-forced). Quarter the apples and remove the cores (leave the skin on). Roughly chop into bite-sized pieces. Place into a large saucepan with the cinnamon, nutmeg, orange zest and ⅓ cup (80 ml) water.
2. Bring to the boil over medium-high heat. Cook for about 10 minutes, stirring often, until the apples are tender and the liquid has evaporated. Pour the cooked apple mixture into a 30 cm × 20 cm (approx.) baking dish and set aside.
3. To make the crumble topping, combine the oats, coconut and olive oil in a bowl and mix together well. Spread the crumble mixture evenly over the apples. Sprinkle with the chopped almonds.
4. Bake for 15–20 minutes, until heated through and golden on top. Serve warm, with a dollop of Greek yoghurt.

Note: You can use any variety of apples, such as pink lady and Granny Smith. Walnuts or macadamias also work well in place of the almonds.

HEALTHIER CARROT CAKE (with video)

A better-for-you version of a classic favourite! This cake is perfect to take for a group gathering and share with family and friends. You can decorate the top of the cake with berries, nuts or whatever you can think of. This cake can also be sliced into portions and frozen if desired, but it is most delicious when enjoyed fresh.

Serves 16

Prep Time: 15 minutes
Cooking Time: 1 hour 15 minutes

1 spiced tea bag (such as chai tea)
1 cup (160 g) sultanas
500 g carrots (about 5), grated
3 eggs, lightly beaten
¼ cup (60 ml) olive oil
¼ cup (90 g) honey
1 teaspoon vanilla extract
2 cups (240 g) ground almonds
1 cup (160 g) wholemeal self-raising flour
2 teaspoons baking powder
1 teaspoon ground cinnamon
½ teaspoon ground nutmeg
1 cup (280 g) plain or vanilla Greek yoghurt, to serve

1. Preheat the oven to 170°C (fan-forced). Lightly grease a 20–22 cm springform cake tin and line the base with baking paper. Stand the tin on a baking tray.
2. Boil the kettle and place the tea bag into a heatproof bowl or jug. Add about 1½ cups boiling water and allow to steep for 3–4 minutes. Remove the tea bag. Add the sultanas to the tea and set aside to soak for 5–10 minutes, until soft. Drain well.
3. Place the carrot into a large mixing bowl and add the soaked sultanas, eggs, olive oil, honey, vanilla, ground almonds, flour, baking powder and spices. Fold together gently until evenly combined. Transfer the batter to the prepared tin and smooth the surface.

4. Bake for 1 hour to 1 hour 15 minutes. The cake is ready when the edges are golden, and the middle is firm to the touch. Set aside to cool in the tin.

5. Remove the cake from the tin and place on a serving plate. Spoon the yoghurt on top of the cake and spread out to cover. Cut into wedges and serve immediately.

Note: If the cake won't all be eaten in one sitting, you could serve the yoghurt on the side.

AFTERWORD: THE GIFT

Raising children can often feel like a tug of war. You want to enjoy your time with them, as conflict free as possible, yet you know that you cannot succumb to their every demand. This is the parental balancing act.

There are many wonderful things that a parent can do for their child. They can buy them the latest iPhone, they can take them on a holiday to the beach, they can provide financial support for their university degree, and they can even help them with a deposit for their first house. These are all kind and generous offerings, but the sum of all of them combined does not equate to the gift of true health.

You are the key to your child's health. They will learn the foundations of health almost entirely through what they observe in you and the food experience you provide for them throughout their childhood.

There are libraries full of books that scientifically explain the physical, physiological and mental impacts of poor health choices versus healthy ones. These choices commence in the womb and continue right through to adulthood, and you, as the parent, have the opportunity to set your child on the right path, to set them up for life while improving your own health along the way. I hope this book, and the whole family approach, will help you do that.

At its best moments, being a parent is the greatest joy of all. It is a gift that the universe has given to you. The best way for you to return this gift is to be an example that steers your child to a lifetime of positive health.

REFERENCES

Introduction

Clemente-Suárez, V. J. et al. (2023). 'Global impacts of western diet and its effects on metabolism and health: A narrative review.' *Nutrients*, 15(12): 2749.

Georgieff, M. K. (2023). 'Early life nutrition and brain development: breakthroughs, challenges and new horizons.' *Proceedings of the Nutrition Society*, 82(2): 104–12.

Machado, P. P. et al. (2020). 'Ultra-processed food consumption and obesity in the Australian adult population.' *Nutrition and Diabetes*, 10(1): 39.

Prado, E. L. and K. G. Dewey (2014). 'Nutrition and brain development in early life.' *Nutrition Reviews*, 72(4): 267–84.

Purnell, J. Q. and C. W. le Roux (2024). 'Hypothalamic control of body fat mass by food intake: The key to understanding why obesity should be treated as a disease.' *Diabetes Obesity and Metabolism*, 26(2): 3–12.

Willett, W. C. (2012). 'Dietary fats and coronary heart disease.' *Journal of Internal Medicine*, 272(1): 13–24.

Zheng, M. B. et al. (2024). 'Editorial: Exploring obesity risk, prevention and research innovation in the first 2000 days of life, volume II.' *Frontiers in Endocrinology*, 15.

Chapter 1

Askie, L. M. et al. (2020). 'Interventions commenced by early infancy to prevent child-hood obesity – The EPOCH Collaboration: An individual participant data prospective meta-analysis of four randomised controlled trials.' *Pediatric Obesity*, 15(6).

Aune, D. et al. (2017). 'Fruit and vegetable intake and the risk of cardiovascular disease, total cancer and all-cause mortality – a systematic review and dose-response meta-analysis of prospective studies.' *International Journal of Epidemiology*, 46(3): 1029–56.

Bucchianeri, M. M. et al. (2013). 'Weightism, racism, classism, and sexism: Shared forms of harassment in adolescents.' *Journal of Adolescent Health*, 53(1): 47–53.

Chen, Y. T. et al. (2021). 'Associations of early pregnancy BMI with adverse pregnancy outcomes and infant neurocognitive development.' *Scientific Reports*, 11(1): 3793.

Dietitians of Canada et al. (2004). 'The use of growth charts for assessing and monitoring growth in Canadian infants and children.' *Canadian Journal of Dietetic Practice and Research*, 65(1): 22–32.

Espelage, D. L. et al. (2014). 'Teacher and staff perceptions of school environment as predictors of student aggression, victimisation, and willingness to intervene in bullying situations.' *School Psychology Quarterly*, 29(3): 287–305.

Fernández-Elías, V. E. et al. (2015). 'Relationship between muscle water and glycogen recovery after prolonged exercise in the heat in humans.' *European Journal of Applied Physiology*, 115(9): 1919–26.

Greenway, F. L. (2015). 'Physiological adaptations to weight loss and factors favouring weight regain.' *International Journal of Obesity*, 39(8): 1188–96.

Hills, A. P. et al. (2023). 'Body composition from birth to 2 years.' *European Journal of Clinical Nutrition*.

Holland, G. and M. Tiggemann (2016). 'A systematic review of the impact of the use of social networking sites on body image and disordered eating outcomes.' *Body Image*, 17: 100–10.

Johnston, L. B. et al. (2002). 'Genetic factors contributing to birth weight.' *Archives of Disease in Childhood – Fetal and Neonatal Edition*, 86(1): F2–3.

Kuk, J. L. et al. (2023). 'Changes in the prevalence of US adults using diet, exercise, pharmaceuticals and diet products for weight loss over time: Analysis of NHANES 1999–2018.' *PLoS One*, 18(10).

Lessard, L. M. and R. M. Puhl (2021). 'Reducing educators' weight bias: The role of school-based anti-bullying policies.' *Journal of School Health*, 91(10): 796–801.

Loos, R. J. F. and G. S. H. Yeo (2022). 'The genetics of obesity: From discovery to biology.' *Nature Reviews Genetics*, 23(2): 120–33.

Loth, K. et al. (2014). 'Food-related parenting practices and child and adolescent weight and weight-related behaviours.' *Clinical Practice (London, England)*, 11(2): 207–20.

Lydecker, J. A. et al. (2018). 'Associations of parents' self, child, and other "fat talk" with child eating behaviours and weight.' *International Journal of Eating Disorders*, 51(6): 527–34.

Magnus, P. (1984). 'Causes of variation in birth-weight – a study of offspring of twins.' *Clinical Genetics*, 25(1): 15–24.

Mahmoud, R. et al. (2022). 'Genetics of obesity in humans: A clinical review.' *International Journal of Molecular Sciences*, 23(19): 11005.

Mozaffarian, D. et al. (2011). 'Changes in diet and lifestyle and long-term weight gain in women and men.' *New England Journal of Medicine*, 364(25): 2392–404.

Müller, M. J. et al. (2010). 'Is there evidence for a set point that regulates human body weight?' *F1000 Medicine Reports*, 2: 59.

Pietiläinen, K. H. et al. (2012). 'Does dieting make you fat? A twin study.' *International Journal of Obesity*, 36(3): 456–64.

Qi, Q. et al. (2014). 'Fried food consumption, genetic risk, and body mass index: Gene-diet interaction analysis in three US cohort studies.' *BMJ – British Medical Journal*, 348.

Rahman, A. et al. (2018). 'How often parents make decisions with their children is associated with obesity.' *BMC Pediatrics*, 18(1): 311.

Rebello, C. J. et al. (2022). 'Low-energy dense potato- and bean-based diets reduce body weight and insulin resistance: A randomised, feeding, equivalence trial.' *Journal of Medicinal Food*, 25(12): 1155–63.

Schneider, H. J. et al. (2010). 'The predictive value of different measures of obesity for incident cardiovascular events and mortality.' *Journal of Clinical Endocrinology and Metabolism*, 95(4): 1777–85.

Simmonds, M. et al. (2016). 'Predicting adult obesity from childhood obesity: A systematic review and meta-analysis.' *Obesity Reviews*, 17(2): 95–107.

Sironi, A. M. et al. (2012). 'Impact of increased visceral and cardiac fat on cardiometabolic risk and disease.' *Diabetic Medicine*, 29(5): 622–7.

Versele, V. et al. (2022). 'The influence of parental body composition and lifestyle on offspring growth trajectories.' *Pediatric Obesity*, 17(10).

Wills, B. (1987). 'Dieting in adolescence.' *New Zealand Medical Journal*, 100(816): 31.

Zhang, J. et al. (2023). 'Pre-pregnancy body mass index has greater influence on newborn weight and perinatal outcome than weight control during pregnancy in obese women.' *Archives of Public Health*, 81(1): 5.

Zheng, M. B. et al. (2024). 'Editorial: Exploring obesity risk, prevention and research innovation in the first 2000 days of life, volume II.' *Frontiers in Endocrinology*, 15.

Zong, X. N. et al. (2022). 'Maternal pre-pregnancy body mass index categories and infant birth outcomes: A population-based study of 9 million mother-infant pairs.' *Frontiers in Nutrition*, 9.

Chapter 2

Anzman-Frasca, S. et al. (2012). 'Repeated exposure and associative conditioning promote preschool children's liking of vegetables.' *Appetite*, 58(2): 543–53.

Behrens, M. and W. Meyerhof (2006). 'Bitter taste receptors and human bitter taste perception.' *Cellular and Molecular Life Sciences*, 63(13): 1501–9.

Borowitz, S. M. (2021). 'First bites – why, when and what solid foods to feed infants.' *Frontiers in Pediatrics*, 9: 654171.

Carruth, B. R. et al. (2004). 'Prevalence of picky eaters among infants and toddlers and their caregivers' decisions about offering a new food.' *Journal of the American Dietetic Association*, 104(1): s57–64.

Daniels, L. A. et al. (2015). 'An early feeding practices intervention for obesity prevention.' *Pediatrics*, 136(1): e40–9.

De Cosmi, V. et al. (2017). 'Early taste experiences and later food choices.' *Nutrients*, 9(2): 107.

Drewnowski, A. and C. Gomez-Carneros (2000). 'Bitter taste, phytonutrients and the consumer: A review.' *American Journal of Clinical Nutrition*, 72(6): 1424–35.

Ester, T. and S. Kullmann (2022). 'Neurobiological regulation of eating behaviour: Evidence based on non-invasive brain stimulation.' *Reviews in Endocrine and Metabolic Disorders*, 23(4): 753–72.

Galloway, A. T. et al. (2006). '"Finish your soup": Counterproductive effects of pressuring children to eat on intake and affect.' *Appetite*, 46(3): 318–23.

Gibson, E. L. and L. Cooke (2017). 'Understanding food fussiness and its implications for food choice, health, weight and interventions in young children: The impact of Professor Jane Wardle.' *Current Obesity Reports*, 6(1): 46–56.

Harris, G. (2008). 'Development of taste and food preferences in children.' *Current Opinion in Clinical Nutrition and Metabolic Care*, 11(3): 315–99.

Jansen, P. W. et al. (2020). 'Associations of parents' use of food as reward with children's eating behaviour and BMI in a population-based cohort.' *Pediatric Obesity*, 15(11).

Kähkönen, K. et al. (2018). 'Sensory-based food education in early childhood education and care, willingness to choose and eat fruit and vegetables, and the moderating role of maternal education and food neophobia.' *Public Health Nutrition*, 21(13): 2443–53.

Lally, P. et al. (2010). 'How are habits formed: Modelling habit formation in the real world.' *European Journal of Social Psychology*, 40(6): 998–1009.

Loth, K. et al. (2014). 'Food-related parenting practices and child and adolescent weight and weight-related behaviours.' *Clinical Practice (London, England)*, 11(2): 207–20.

Mallan, K. M. et al. (2016). 'The relationship between number of fruits, vegetables and noncore foods tried at age 14 months and food preferences, dietary intake patterns, fussy eating behaviour and weight status at age 3.7 years.' *Journal of the Academy of Nutrition and Dietetics*, 116(4): 630–7.

Mallan, K. M. et al. (2018). 'Feeding a fussy eater: Examining longitudinal bidirectional relationships between child fussy eating and maternal feeding practices.' *Journal of Pediatric Psychology*, 43(10): 1138–46.

Melgar-Locatelli, S. et al. (2023). 'Nutrition and adult neurogenesis in the hippocampus: Does what you eat help you remember?' *Frontiers in Neuroscience*, 17.

Nix, R. L. et al. (2021). 'Improving toddlers' healthy eating habits and self-regulation: A randomised controlled trial.' *Pediatrics*, 147(1).

Reed, D. R. and A. Knaapila (2010). 'Genetics of taste and smell: Poisons and pleasures.' *Genes and Obesity*. C. Bouchard. 94: 213–40.

Rigal, N. et al. (2016). 'Is harsh caregiving effective in toddlers with low inhibitory control? An experimental study in the food domain.' *Infant Behaviour and Development*, 43: 5–12.

Rubio, B. et al. (2008). 'Measuring willingness to try new foods: A self-report questionnaire for French-speaking children.' *Appetite*, 50(2–3): 408–14.

Scaglioni, S. et al. (2018). 'Factors influencing children's eating behaviours.' *Nutrients*, 10(6): 706.

Wiles, N. J. et al. (2009). '"Junk food" diet and childhood behavioural problems: Results from the ALSPAC cohort.' *European Journal of Clinical Nutrition*, 63(4): 491–8.

Chapter 3

Arima, Y. and H. Fukuoka (2020). 'Developmental origins of health and disease theory in cardiology.' *Journal of Cardiology*, 76(1): 14–7.

Bandín, C. et al. (2015). 'Meal timing affects glucose tolerance, substrate oxidation and circadian-related variables: A randomised, crossover trial.' *International Journal of Obesity (London)*, 39(5): 828–33.

Bhupathi, V. et al. (2020). 'Dairy intake and risk of cardiovascular disease.' *Current Cardiology Reports*, 22(3): 11.

Bo, S. et al. (2015). 'Is the timing of caloric intake associated with variation in diet-induced thermogenesis and in the metabolic pattern? A randomised cross-over study.' *International Journal Obesity (London)* 39(12): 1689–95.

Bucher, H. C. et al. (1996). 'Effect of calcium supplementation on pregnancy-induced hypertension and pre-eclampsia: A meta-analysis of randomised controlled trials.' *JAMA*, 275(14): 1113–7.

Cichero, J. A. Y. (2016). 'Introducing solid foods using baby-led weaning vs. spoon-feeding: A focus on oral development, nutrient intake and quality of research to bring balance to the debate.' *Nutrition Bulletin*, 41(1): 72–7.

Cusick, S. E. and M. K. Georgieff (2016). 'The role of nutrition in brain development: The golden opportunity of the "first 1000 days".' *Journal of Pediatrics*, 175: 16–21.

Daniels, L. A. et al. (2009). 'The NOURISH randomised control trial: Positive feeding practices and food preferences in early childhood – a primary prevention program for childhood obesity.' *BMC Public Health*, 9: 387.

Daniels, L. A. et al. (2015). 'An early feeding practices intervention for obesity prevention.' *Pediatrics*, 136(1): e40–9.

Dawber, T. R. et al. (1982). 'Eggs, serum cholesterol and coronary heart disease.' *American Journal Clinical Nutrition*, 36(4): 617–25.

De Cosmi, V. et al. (2017). 'Early taste experiences and later food choices.' *Nutrients*, 9(2): 107.

De Sanctis, V. et al. (2021). 'Early and long-term consequences of nutritional stunting: From childhood to adulthood.' *Acta Biomed*, 92(1): e2021168.

Díaz-López, A. et al. (2024). 'Close adherence to a mediterranean diet during pregnancy decreases childhood overweight/obesity: A prospective study.' *Nutrients*, 16(4).

DiNicolantonio, J. J. and J. H. O'Keefe (2018). 'Importance of maintaining a low omega-6/omega-3 ratio for reducing inflammation.' *Open Heart*, 5(2): e000946.

Dovey, T. M. et al. (2008). 'Food neophobia and "picky/fussy" eating in children: A review.' *Appetite*, 50(2–3): 181–93.

Du Toit, G. et al. (2015). 'Randomised trial of peanut consumption in infants at risk for peanut allergy.' *New England Journal of Medicine*, 372(9): 803–13.

Du Toit, G. et al. (2016). 'Effect of avoidance on peanut allergy after early peanut consumption.' *New England Journal of Medicine*, 374(15): 1435–43.

Duan, Y. et al. (2018). 'Inflammatory links between high fat diets and diseases.' *Front Immunology*, 9: 2649.

Duarte, C. et al. (2021). 'Dairy versus other saturated fats source and cardiometabolic risk markers: Systematic review of randomised controlled trials.' *Critical Reviews in Food Science and Nutrition*, 61(3): 450–61.

Fehm, H. L. et al. (2006). 'The selfish brain: Competition for energy resources.' *Progress in Brain Research*, 153: 129–40.

Feng, Y. et al. (2022). 'Consumption of dairy products and the risk of overweight or obesity, hypertension, and type 2 diabetes mellitus: A dose-response meta-analysis and systematic review of cohort studies.' *Advances in Nutrition*, 13(6): 2165–79.

Flores, T. R. et al. (2024). 'Pre-pregnancy maternal BMI and trajectories of BMI-for-age in children up to four years of age: Findings from the 2015 Pelotas (Brazil) birth cohort.' *International Journal of Obesity (London)*, 48(3): 353–9.

Foster, G. D. et al. (2003). 'A randomised trial of a low-carbohydrate diet for obesity.' *New England Journal of Medicine*, 348(21): 2082–90.

Fuller, N. R. et al. (2015). 'Egg consumption and human cardio-metabolic health in people with and without diabetes.' *Nutrients*, 7(9): 7399–420.

Georgoulis, M. et al. (2023). 'Sustained improvements in the cardiometabolic profile of patients with obstructive sleep apnea after a weight-loss Mediterranean diet/lifestyle intervention: 12-month follow-up (6 months post-intervention) of the "MIMOSA" randomised clinical trial.' *Nutrition, Metabolism and Cardiovascular Diseases*, 33(5): 1019–28.

Gholami, F. et al. (2017). 'The effect of dairy consumption on the prevention of cardiovascular diseases: A meta-analysis of prospective studies.' *Journal of Cardiovascular and Thoracic Research*, 9(1): 1–11.

Hall, N. Y. et al. (2024). 'Global prevalence of adolescent use of nonprescription weight-loss products.' *JAMA Network Open*, 7(1).

Hansen, C. D. et al. (2023). 'Effect of calorie-unrestricted low-carbohydrate, high-fat diet versus high-carbohydrate, low-fat diet on type 2 diabetes and nonalcoholic fatty liver disease : A randomised controlled trial.' *Annals of Internal Medicine*, 176(1): 10–21.

Hebebrand, J. et al. (2014). '"Eating addiction", rather than "food addiction", better captures addictive-like eating behaviour.' *Neuroscience and Biobehavioural Reviews*, 47: 295–306.

Heymsfield, S. B. et al. (2024). 'Proportion of caloric restriction-induced weight loss as skeletal muscle.' *Obesity (Silver Spring)*, 32(1): 32–40.

Hidaka, N. et al. (2023). 'Effect of mastication evaluation and intervention on body composition and biochemical indices in female patients with obesity: A randomised controlled trial.' *BMC Endocrine Disorders*, 23(1): 134.

Ho, S. et al. (2014). 'Comparative effects of A1 versus A2 beta-casein on gastrointestinal measures: A blinded randomised cross-over pilot study.' *European Journal of Clinical Nutrition*, 68(9): 994–1000.

Ierodiakonou, D. et al. (2016). 'Timing of allergenic food introduction to the infant diet and risk of allergic or autoimmune disease: A systematic review and meta-analysis.' *JAMA*, 316(11): 1181–92.

Islam, M. A. et al. (2019). 'Trans fatty acids and lipid profile: A serious risk factor to cardiovascular disease, cancer and diabetes.' *Diabetes and Metabolic Syndrome*, 13(2): 1643–7.

Jacka, F. N. et al. (2015). 'Western diet is associated with a smaller hippocampus: A longitudinal investigation.' *BMC Medicine*, 13: 215.

Jansen, P. W. et al. (2017). 'Bi-directional associations between child fussy eating and parents' pressure to eat: Who influences whom?' *Physiology and Behaviour*, 176: 101–6.

Jarlenski, M. P. et al. (2014). 'Effects of breastfeeding on postpartum weight loss among U.S. women.' *Preventative Medicine*, 69: 146–50.

Jones, S. W. et al. (2020). 'Spoonfeeding is associated with increased infant weight but only amongst formula-fed infants.' *Maternal and Child Nutrition*, 16(3).

Jovanovic, B. (2017). 'Ingestion of microplastics by fish and its potential consequences from a physical perspective.' *Integrated Environmental Assessment and Management*, 13(3): 510–5.

Khan, S. U. et al. (2021). 'Effect of omega-3 fatty acids on cardiovascular outcomes: A systematic review and meta-analysis.' *EClinicalMedicine*, 38: 100997.

Kim, K. et al. (2021). 'Nutritional adequacy and diet quality are associated with standardised height-for-age among U.S. children.' *Nutrients*, 13(5): 1689.

Koeder, C. and F. J. A. Perez-Cueto (2024). 'Vegan nutrition: A preliminary guide for health professionals.' *Critical Reviews in Food Science and Nutrition*, 64(3): 670–707.

Kuo, A. A. et al. (2011). 'Introduction of solid food to young infants.' *Maternal and Child Health Journal*, 15(8): 1185–94.

Larbey, C. et al. (2019). 'Cooked starchy food in hearths ca. 120 kya and 65 kya (MIS 5e and MIS 4) from Klasies River Cave, South Africa.' *Journal of Human Evolution*, 131: 210–27.

Lerner, B. A. et al. (2019). 'Going against the grains: Gluten-free diets in patients without coeliac disease – worthwhile or not?' *Digestive Diseases and Sciences*, 64(7): 1740–7.

Leuck, M. et al. (2014). 'Circadian rhythm of energy expenditure and oxygen consumption.' *JPEN. Journal of Parenteral and Enteral Nutrition*, 38(2): 263–8.

Levi, F. et al. (2001). 'Dietary fibre and the risk of colorectal cancer.' *European Journal of Cancer*, 37(16): 2091–6.

López-Sobaler, A. M. et al. (2020). 'Effect of dairy intake with or without energy restriction on body composition of adults: overview of systematic reviews and meta-analyses of randomised controlled trials.' *Nutrition Reviews*, 78(11): 901–13.

Mallan, K. M. et al. (2016). 'The relationship between number of fruits, vegetables, and noncore foods tried at age 14 months and food preferences, dietary intake patterns, fussy eating behaviour and weight status at age 3.7 years.' *Journal of the Academy of Nutrition and Dietetics*, 116(4): 630–7.

Marshall, N. E. et al. (2022). 'The importance of nutrition in pregnancy and lactation: Lifelong consequences.' *American Journal of Obstetrics and Gynecology*, 226(5): 607–32.

Martinez-Gonzalez, M. A. and N. Martin-Calvo (2016). 'Mediterranean diet and life expectancy; beyond olive oil, fruits and vegetables.' *Current Opinion in Clinical Nutrition and Metabolic Care*, 19(6): 401–7.

Milunsky, A. et al. (1989). 'Multivitamin/folic acid supplementation in early pregnancy reduces the prevalence of neural tube defects.' *JAMA*, 262(20): 2847–52.

Mishra, S. et al. (2008). 'Effect of processing on slowly digestible starch and resistant starch in potato.' *Starch-Starke*, 60(9): 500–7.

Nestel, P. J. and T. A. Mori (2022). 'Dairy foods: Is its cardiovascular risk profile changing?' *Current Atherosclerosis Reports*, 24(1): 33–40.

Nguyen, M. et al. (2024). 'Consumption of 100% fruit juice and body weight in children and adults: A systematic review and meta-analysis.' *JAMA Pediatrics*, 178(3): 237–46.

Olsen, S. F. and N. J. Secher (2002). 'Low consumption of seafood in early pregnancy as a risk factor for preterm delivery: Prospective cohort study.' *BMJ*, 324(7335): 447.

Pearce, K. L. et al. (2011). 'Egg consumption as part of an energy-restricted high-protein diet improves blood lipid and blood glucose profiles in individuals with type 2 diabetes.' *British Journal of Nutrition*, 105(4): 584–92.

Purnell, J. Q. and C. W. le Roux (2024). 'Hypothalamic control of body fat mass by food intake: The key to understanding why obesity should be treated as a disease.' *Diabetes Obesity and Metabolism*, 26(2): 3–12.

Qin, L. Q. et al. (2015). 'Dairy consumption and risk of cardiovascular disease: An updated meta-analysis of prospective cohort studies.' *Asia Pacific Journal of Clinical Nutrition*, 24(1): 90–100.

Richter, J. et al. (2020). 'Twice as high diet-induced thermogenesis after breakfast vs dinner on high-calorie as well as low-calorie meals.' *Journal of Clinical Endocrinology Metabolism*, 105(3).

Rodriguez-Martinez, A. et al. (2020). 'Height and body-mass index trajectories of school-aged children and adolescents from 1985 to 2019 in 200 countries and territories: A pooled analysis of 2181 population-based studies with 65 million participants.' *Lancet*, 396(10261): 1511–24.

Saavedra, S. et al. (2022). 'Impact of dietary mercury intake during pregnancy on the health of neonates and children: A systematic review.' *Nutrition Reviews*, 80(2): 317–28.

Sacks, F. M. et al. (2009). 'Comparison of weight-loss diets with different compositions of fat, protein and carbohydrates.' *New England Journal of Medicine*, 360(9): 859–73.

Sato, M. et al. (2011). 'Acute effect of late evening meal on diurnal variation of blood glucose and energy metabolism.' *Obesity Research and Clinical Practice*, 5(3): e169–266.

Sebastiani, G. et al. (2019). 'The effects of vegetarian and vegan diet during pregnancy on the health of mothers and offspring.' *Nutrients*, 11(3): 557.

See, J. A. et al. (2015). 'Practical insights into gluten-free diets.' *Nature Reviews Gastroenterology and Hepatology*, 12(10): 580–91.

Sezaki, A. et al. (2022). 'Association between the mediterranean diet score and healthy life expectancy: A global comparative study.' *Journal of Nutrition, Health and Aging*, 26(6): 621–7.

Shipp, G. M. et al. (2024). 'Maternal pre-pregnancy BMI, breastfeeding, and child BMI.' *Pediatrics*, 153(1).

Siri-Tarino, P. W. et al. (2010). 'Meta-analysis of prospective cohort studies evaluating the association of saturated fat with cardiovascular disease.' *American Journal of Clinical Nutrition*, 91(3): 535–46.

Siri-Tarino, P. W. et al. (2010). 'Saturated fatty acids and risk of coronary heart disease: modulation by replacement nutrients.' *Current Atherosclerosis Reports*, 12(6): 384–90.

Skov, A. R. et al. (1999). 'Randomised trial on protein vs carbohydrate in ad libitum fat reduced diet for the treatment of obesity.' *International Journal of Obesity and Related Metabolic Disorders*, 23(5): 528–36.

Sood, S. et al. (2022). 'Higher adherence to a Mediterranean diet is associated with improved insulin sensitivity and selected markers of inflammation in individuals who are overweight and obese without diabetes.' *Nutrients*, 14(20): 4437.

Staudacher, H. M. and P. R. Gibson (2015). 'How healthy is a gluten-free diet?' *British Journal of Nutrition*, 114(10): 1539–41.

Taetzsch, A. et al. (2018). 'Are gluten-free diets more nutritious? An evaluation of self-selected and recommended gluten-free and gluten-containing dietary patterns.' *Nutrients*, 10(12): 1881.

Taylor, C. M. et al. (2015). 'Picky/fussy eating in children: Review of definitions, assessment, prevalence and dietary intakes.' *Appetite*, 95: 349–59.

Totzauer, M. et al. (2022). 'Different protein intake in the first year and its effects on adiposity rebound and obesity throughout childhood: 11 years follow-up of a randomised controlled trial.' *Pediatric Obesity*, 17(12).

Trogen, B. et al. (2022). 'Early introduction of allergenic foods and the prevention of food allergy.' *Nutrients*, 14(13).

Uauy, R. and A. Valenzuela (2000). 'Marine oils: the health benefits of n-3 fatty acids.' *Nutrition*, 16(7–8): 680–4.

Waagaard, L. et al. (2023). 'Body mass index and weight gain in pregnancy and cardiovascular health in middle age: A cohort study.' *BJOG*.

Wiles, N. J. et al. (2009). '"Junk food" diet and childhood behavioural problems: Results from the ALSPAC cohort.' *European Journal of Clinical Nutrition*, 63(4): 491–8.

Zaragoza-Martí, A. et al. (2022). 'Adherence to the Mediterranean diet in pregnancy and its benefits on maternal-fetal health: A systematic review of the literature.' *Frontiers in Nutrition*, 9: 813942.

Zheng, M. et al. (2024). 'Breastfeeding and the longitudinal changes of body mass index in childhood and adulthood: A systematic review.' *Advances in Nutrition*, 15(1): 100152.

Chapter 4

Anzman-Frasca, S. et al. (2012). 'Repeated exposure and associative conditioning promote preschool children's liking of vegetables.' *Appetite*, 58(2): 543–53.

Benton, D. (2004). 'Role of parents in the determination of the food preferences of children and the development of obesity.' *International Journal of Obesity*, 28(7): 858–69.

Birch, L. L. (1999). 'Development of food preferences.' *Annual Review of Nutrition*, 19: 41–62.

Birch, L. L. and M. Deysher (1986). 'Caloric compensation and sensory specific satiety: evidence for self regulation of food intake by young children.' *Appetite*, 7(4): 323–31.

Boeing, H. et al. (2012). 'Critical review: vegetables and fruit in the prevention of chronic diseases.' *European Journal of Nutrition*, 51(6): 637–63.

Brown, R. and J. Ogden (2004). 'Children's eating attitudes and behaviour: a study of the modelling and control theories of parental influence.' *Health Education Research*, 19(3): 261–71.

Carruth, B. R. et al. (2004). 'Prevalence of picky eaters among infants and toddlers and their caregivers' decisions about offering a new food.' *Journal of the American Dietetic Association*, 104(1): S57–S64.

Cinotto, S. (2006). '"Everyone would be around the table": American family meal-times in historical perspective, 1850–1960.' *New Directions for Child and Adolescent Development*, (111): 17–34.

Coulthard, H. and D. Thakker (2015). 'Enjoyment of tactile play is associated with lower food neophobia in preschool children.' *Journal of the Academy of Nutrition and Dietetics*, 115(7): 1134–40.

De Cosmi, V. et al. (2017). 'Early taste experiences and later food choices.' *Nutrients*, 9(2).

Fabiansson, S. U. (2006). 'Precision in nutritional information declarations on food labels in Australia.' *Asia Pacific Journal of Clinical Nutrition*, 15(4): 451–8.

Galloway, A. T., et al. (2006). '"Finish your soup": Counterproductive effects of pressuring children to eat on intake and affect.' *Appetite*, 46(3): 318–23.

Harris, G. (2008). 'Development of taste and food preferences in children.' *Current Opinion in Clinical Nutrition and Metabolic Care*, 11(3): 315–9.

Kähkönen, K. et al. (2018). 'Sensory-based food education in early childhood education and care, willingness to choose and eat fruit and vegetables, and the moderating role of maternal education and food neophobia.' *Public Health Nutrition*, 21(13): 2443–53.

Mallan, K. M. et al. (2018). 'Feeding a fussy eater: examining longitudinal bidirectional relationships between child fussy eating and maternal feeding practices.' *Journal of Pediatric Psychology*, 43(10): 1138–46.

Melgar-Locatelli, S. et al. (2023). 'Nutrition and adult neurogenesis in the hippocampus: Does what you eat help you remember?' *Frontiers in Neuroscience*, 17.

Pliner, P. and C. Stallberg-White (2000). '"Pass the ketchup, please": familiar flavors increase children's willingness to taste novel foods.' *Appetite*, 34(1): 95–103.

Richter, J. et al. (2020). 'Twice as high diet-induced thermogenesis after break-fast vs dinner on high-calorie as well as low-calorie meals.' *Journal of Clinical Endocrinology and Metabolism*, 105(3).

Rigal, N. et al. (2016). 'Is harsh caregiving effective in toddlers with low inhibi-tory control? An experimental study in the food domain.' *Infant Behaviour and Development*, 43: 5–12.

Rubio, B. et al. (2008). 'Measuring willingness to try new foods: A self-report question-naire for French-speaking children.' *Appetite*, 50(2–3): 408–14.

Scaglioni, S. et al. (2018). 'Factors influencing children's eating behaviours.' *Nutrients*, 10(6): 706.

Chapter 5

Blundell, J. E. et al. (2015). 'Appetite control and energy balance: Impact of exercise.' *Obesity Reviews*, 16(1): 67–76.

Kohl, H. W. et al. (2012). 'The pandemic of physical inactivity: Global action for public health.' *Lancet*, 380(9838): 294–305.

Martins, C. et al. (2008). 'A review of the effects of exercise on appetite regulation: An obesity perspective.' *International Journal of Obesity*, 32(9): 1337–47.

May, L. E. et al. (2023). 'Influence of supervised maternal aerobic exercise during pregnancy on one-month-old neonatal cardiac function and outflow: A pilot study.' *Medicine and Science in Sports and Exercise*, 55(11): 1977–84.

Oygur, I. et al. (2021). *The Lived Experience of Child-Owned Wearables: Comparing Children's and Parents' Perspectives on Activity Tracking*. CHI Conference on Human Factors in Computing Systems, Electrical Network.

Perales, M. et al. (2017). 'Exercise during pregnancy.' *JAMA – Journal of the American Medical Association*, 317(11): 1113–4.

Chapter 6

Brown, T. T. and T. L. Jernigan (2012). 'Brain development during the preschool years.' *Neuropsychology Review*, 22(4): 313–33.

Budday, S. et al. (2015). 'Physical biology of human brain development.' *Frontiers in Cellular Neuroscience*, 9: 257.

Clark, I. and H. P. Landolt (2017). 'Coffee, caffeine and sleep: A systematic review of epidemiological studies and randomised controlled trials.' *Sleep Medicine Reviews*, 31: 70–8.

Ebrahim, I. O. et al. (2013). 'Alcohol and sleep I: Effects on normal sleep.' *Alcoholism – Clinical and Experimental Research*, 37(4): 539–49.

van Egmond, L. T. et al. (2023). 'Effects of acute sleep loss on leptin, ghrelin and adiponectin in adults with healthy weight and obesity: A laboratory study.' *Obesity (Silver Spring)*, 31(3): 635–41.

Fuhrmann, D. et al. (2015). 'Adolescence as a sensitive period of brain development.' *Trends in Cognitive Sciences*, 19(10): 558–66.

Fatima, Y. et al. (2020). 'Late bedtime and body mass index gain in Indigenous Australian children in the longitudinal study of indigenous children.' *Acta Paediatrica*, 109(10): 2084–90.

Goetz, A. R. et al. (2022). 'The roles of sleep and eating patterns in adiposity gain among preschool-aged children.' *American Journal of Clinical Nutrition*, 116(5): 1334–42.

Guerrero, M. D. et al. (2019). 'Screen time and problem behaviours in children: Exploring the mediating role of sleep duration.' *International Journal of Behavioural Nutrition and Physical Activity*, 16(1): 105.

Li, M. et al. (2024). 'Causal relationships between screen use, reading and brain development in early adolescents.' *Advanced Science (Weinh)*, 11(11): e2307540.

Nagata, J. M. et al. (2023). 'Contemporary screen time modalities and disruptive behaviour disorders in children: A prospective cohort study.' *Journal of Child Psychology and Psychiatry*, 64(1): 125–35.

Nagata, J. M. et al. (2022). 'Screen time use among US adolescents during the COVID-19 pandemic findings from the Adolescent Brain Cognitive Development (ABCD) Study.' *JAMA Pediatrics*, 176(1): 94–6.

Nagata, J. M. et al. (2023). 'Bedtime screen use behaviours and sleep outcomes: Findings from the Adolescent Brain Cognitive Development (ABCD) Study.' *Sleep Health*, 9(4): 497–502.

Neophytou, E. et al. (2021). 'Effects of excessive screen time on neurodevelopment, learning, memory, mental health and neurodegeneration: A scoping review.' *International Journal of Mental Health and Addiction*, 19(3): 724–44.

Paulich, K. N. et al. (2021). 'Screen time and early adolescent mental health, academic and social outcomes in 9- and 10-year-old children: Utilizing the Adolescent Brain Cognitive Development (ABCD) Study.' *PloS One*, 16(9).

Paulus, M. P. et al. (2019). 'Screen media activity and brain structure in youth: Evidence for diverse structural correlation networks from the ABCD Study.' *NeuroImage*, 185: 140–53.

Rihm, J. S. et al. (2019). 'Sleep deprivation selectively upregulates an amygdala-hypothalamic circuit involved in food reward.' *Journal of Neuroscience*, 39(5): 888–99.

Roberston, L. et al. (2022). 'Associations between screen time and internalising disorder diagnoses among 9- to 10-year-olds.' *Journal of Affective Disorders*, 311: 530–7.

Wahl, S. et al. (2019). 'The inner clock – blue light sets the human rhythm.' *Journal of Biophotonics*, 12(12).

West, K. E. et al. (2011). 'Blue light from light-emitting diodes elicits a dose-dependent suppression of melatonin in humans.' *Journal of Applied Physiology*, 110(3): 619–26.

ACKNOWLEDGEMENTS

Without health, you have nothing.

A book only comes to life by being read, so thank you for reading this one. This book took an immense amount of time – a work in progress for the past five years – and it would not have been possible without the invaluable contributions of several incredibly thoughtful, supportive and loving people.

Firstly, to my wife, Sally Rawsthorne. Thank you for always being there for me and for all the work you have put into reading and editing this book. You are the first person who reads my words and the first to tell me what is and isn't working. Your incredible editorial ability really did help bring this all together. I am blessed to have such a loving, intelligent and beautiful person in my life. And without you, I would not be able to do everything I set out to achieve.

To my two beautiful boys, Jude and Jonas. Watching you grow up and experience the world and conquer obstacles as you do it is truly astonishing. The fun has just begun!

To my mother, Diane Fuller, and my brother, Andrew Fuller. You have helped me in so many ways over the years and I am blessed to have such a loving, helpful and kind-hearted mother and brother. You have always been very supportive and generous with your time, which enables me to do things such as write a book.

To my late father, Chris Fuller. You inspired me to work hard, to always put my work into words, and to teach and help others. You will forever be in my thoughts.

To all those people in my life who have helped me in many ways – particularly Ed White, Chris Wilkins and Matt Mooney. I am very thankful for all your help over the years and I truly value your friendship. Ed, you have given me so much of your time and I appreciate your wise words that helped shape this book. The camels may not have made the final edit, but many other things did. Special thanks also to Anna He for her skills in creative content and design, and to Chelsea Hendy for her work on the recipes.

To my publisher, Penguin Random House Australia. This book is, of course, not possible without your support and belief in me, particularly Nikki Christer and Sophie Ambrose, and most recently Brandon VanOver. Sophie, thank you for believing in me from the very start; your wisdom and professionalism have helped bring this message and now series of books to life – I can't believe this is book number four! Thank you for everything you've done. And to Shané Oosthuizen, for your wonderful work helping edit this book. It's been an absolute delight working with you.

There is also the community of people following the IWL plan that I'd like to acknowledge. The continued development of this important message on health – now for the next generation – would not be possible without you, particularly those who have helped co-design the Interval Weight Loss app so that additional support tools are available for adults to regain control of their health and weight. There is an exhaustive list of people who have helped over the years but special mention to Betty Reichstein, Elizabeth Tan, Judith Hooley, Mandy Johnston, Fran Bush, Melinda Di Silvio, Natalie Watson, Steph De Sousa, Sandra Desborough,

Sharon Contin, Brenton Johnson, Ben Lindsay, Chris White, Tim Wallace, Lorraine Bradwell, Nina Demonteverde, Angus Klem and Aisling Fleury.

Lastly, I'd like to acknowledge Professor Tania Markovic, who has inspired me with her intellect and her wisdom, and who has supported me every step of the way. I am truly grateful for all she has done for me at the University of Sydney and Royal Prince Alfred Hospital.

I'd also like to thank Professor Ian Caterson and Professor Stephen Twigg, who have both had a hugely positive impact on my work, and on my career within the University.

Powered by Penguin

Looking for more great reads, exclusive content and book giveaways?

Subscribe to our weekly newsletter.

Scan the QR code or visit penguin.com.au/signup